Barrett's Esophagus and Cancer

Guest Editor

PRATEEK SHARMA, MD

SURGICAL ONCOLOGY CLINICS OF NORTH AMERICA

www.surgonc.theclinics.com

Consulting Editor
NICHOLAS J. PETRELLI, MD

July 2009 • Volume 18 • Number 3

SAUNDERS an imprint of ELSEVIER, Inc.

W.B. SAUNDERS COMPANY
A Division of Elsevier Inc.

1600 John F. Kennedy Boulevard • Suite 1800 • Philadelphia, PA 19103-2899

http://www.theclinics.com

SURGICAL ONCOLOGY CLINICS OF NORTH AMERICA Volume 18, Number 3
July 2009 ISSN 1055-3207, ISBN-13: 978-1-4377-0548-5, ISBN-10: 1-4377-0548-0

Editor: Catherine Bewick
Developmental Editor: Donald Mumford

Surgical Oncology Clinics of North America (ISSN 1055-3207) is published quarterly by Elsevier Inc., 360 Park Avenue South, New York, NY 10010-1710. Months of publication are January, April, July, and October. Business and editorial offices: 1600 John F. Kennedy Boulevard, Suite 1800, Philadelphia, PA 19103-2899. Customer service office: 11830 Westline Industrial Drive, St. Louis, MO 63146. Periodicals postage paid at New York, NY, and additional mailing offices. Subscription prices are $218.00 per year (US individuals), $333.00 (US institutions) $110.00 (US student/resident), $251.00 (Canadian individuals), $414.00 (Canadian institutions), $158.00 (Canadian student/resident), $314.00 (foreign individuals), $414.00 (foreign institutions), and $158.00 (foreign student/ resident). Foreign air speed delivery is included in all *Clinics* subscription prices. All prices are subject to change without notice. POST-MASTER: Send address changes to *Surgical Oncology Clinics of North America,* Elsevier Journals Customer Service, 11830 Westline Industrial Drive, St. Louis, MO 63146. **Customer Service: 1-800-654-2452 (US). From outside the United States, call 314-453-7041. Fax: 314-453-5170. E-mail: JournalsCustomerService-usa@elsevier.com (for print support); JournalsOnlineSupport-usa@elsevier. com (for online support).**

Reprints. For copies of 100 or more, of articles in this publication, please contact the Commercial Reprints Department, Elsevier Inc., 360 Park Avenue South, New York, New York 10010-1710. Tel. 212-633-3813; Fax: 212-462-1935; E-mail: reprints@elsevier.com.

Surgical Oncology Clinics of North America is covered in *MEDLINE/PubMed (Index Medicus)* and *EMBASE/ Excerpta Medica, Current Contents/Clinical Medicine,* and *ISI/BIOMED.*

Printed and bound by CPI Group (UK) Ltd, Croydon, CR0 4YY

Transferred to Digital Print 2011

Contributors

CONSULTING EDITOR

NICHOLAS J. PETRELLI, MD
Bank of America Endowed Medical Director, Helen F. Graham Cancer Center at Christiana Care Health System, Newark, Delaware; Professor of Surgery, Thomas Jefferson University, Philadelphia, Pennsylvania

GUEST EDITOR

PRATEEK SHARMA, MD
Professor of Medicine, Director of Gastrointestinal Fellowship Program, University of Kansas School of Medicine Medical Center, Kansas City, Missouri

AUTHORS

MARIAGNESE BARBERA, PhD
Program Development Fellow, Hutchison-MRC Research Centre, Cambridge, United Kingdom

RAQUEL DAVILA, MD
Division of Gastroenterology, VA North Texas Healthcare System; Assistant Professor of Medicine, University of Texas Southwestern Medical Center at Dallas, Dallas, Texas

GARY W. FALK, MD, MS
Department of Gastroenterology and Hepatology, Center for Swallowing and Esophageal Disorders, Cleveland Clinic; Professor of Medicine, Cleveland Clinic, Lerner College of Medicine of Case Western Reserve University, Cleveland, Ohio

REBECCA C. FITZGERALD, MA (Cantab), MD, FRCP
Group Leader, MRC Cancer Cell Unit, Hutchison-MRC Research Centre; Honorary Consultant, Department of Gastroenterology, Addenbrooke's Hospital; Honorary Consultant, Department of General Medicine, Addenbrooke's Hospital, Cambridge, United Kingdom

SÉBASTIEN GILBERT, MD
Assistant Professor, Director, Lung Volume Reduction Surgery, Division of Thoracic and Foregut Surgery, The Heart, Lung, and Esophageal Surgery Institute, University of Pittsburgh Medical Center, Pittsburgh, Pennsylvania

KATHY HORMI-CARVER, PhD
Assistant Professor of Medicine, Division of Gastroenterology, Department of Medicine, VA North Texas Health Care System and the University of Texas Southwestern Medical School, Dallas, Texas

DAVID H. ILSON, MD, PhD
Gastrointestinal Oncology Service, Department of Medicine, Memorial Sloan-Kettering
Cancer Center, New York, New York

BLAIR A. JOBE, MD, FACS
Sampson Family Endowed Associate Professor of Surgery; Director, Esophageal
Research; Director, Esophageal Diagnostics and Therapeutic Endoscopy, Division
of Thoracic and Foregut Surgery, The Heart, Lung, and Esophageal Surgery Institute,
University of Pittsburgh Medical Center, Pittsburgh, Pennsylvania

GEOFFREY Y. KU, MD
Gastrointestinal Oncology Service, Department of Medicine, Memorial Sloan-Kettering
Cancer Center, New York, New York

JAMES D. LUKETICH, MD
Heart, Lung and Esophageal Surgery Institute, University of Pittsburgh Medical Center,
Presbyterian University Hospital, Pittsburgh, Pennsylvania

LIAM MURRAY, MD
Professor of Cancer Epidemiology, Centre for Public Health, The Queen's University
of Belfast, Belfast, United Kingdom

LENA B. PALMER, MD
Clinical Instructor, Division of Gastroenterology and Hepatology, University of North
Carolina Center for Esophageal Diseases and Swallowing, University of North Carolina
School of Medicine, Chapel Hill, North Carolina

IRFAN QURESHI, MD
Heart, Lung and Esophageal Surgery Institute, University of Pittsburgh Medical Center,
Pittsburgh, Pennsylvania

YVONNE ROMERO, MD
Assistant Professor of Medicine, Division of Gastroenterology and Hepatology,
Departments of Medicine and Otorhinolaryngology, Mayo Clinic College of Medicine,
Rochester, Minnesota

RICHARD E. SAMPLINER, MD
Professor of Medicine, Arizona Health Sciences Center, Southern Arizona VA Health
Care System, Tucson, Arizona

NICHOLAS J. SHAHEEN, MD, MPH
Associate Professor, Departments of Medicine and Epidemiology, Schools of Medicine
and Public Health; Director, University of North Carolina Center for Esophageal Diseases
and Swallowing, University of North Carolina School of Medicine, Chapel Hill,
North Carolina

MANISHA SHENDE, MD
Heart, Lung and Esophageal Surgery Institute, University of Pittsburgh Medical Center,
Presbyterian University Hospital, Pittsburgh, Pennsylvania

RHONDA F. SOUZA, MD
Associate Professor of Medicine, Division of Gastroenterology, Department of Medicine, VA North Texas Health Care System and the University of Texas Southwestern Medical School; Harold C. Simmons Comprehensive Cancer Center, University of Texas Southwestern Medical Center at Dallas, Dallas, Texas

STUART JON SPECHLER, MD
Chief, Division of Gastroenterology, VA North Texas Healthcare System; Professor of Medicine, Berta M. and Cecil O. Patterson Chair in Gastroenterology, University of Texas Southwestern Medical Center at Dallas, Dallas, Texas

HERBERT C. WOLFSEN, MD
Consultant, Division of Gastroenterology and Hepatology, Mayo Clinic, Jacksonville, Florida; Professor, Mayo Medical School, Rochester, Minnesota

LISA YERIAN, MD
Assistant Professor of Pathology, Section Head of Surgical Pathology, Director of Heapatobiliary Pathology, Lerner College of Medicine; Department of Anatomic Pathology, Cleveland Clinic, Cleveland, Ohio

Contents

Barrett's esophagus (BE) is a metaplastic premalignant disorder in which the normal stratified squamous epithelium of the lower esophagus is replaced by a columnar lined epithelium with intestinal differentiation. BE generally occurs in the context of chronic gastroesophageal reflux disease and it is the primary risk factor for the development of esophageal adenocarcinoma, with a conversion rate of 0.5% to 1% per annum. The dramatic increase of esophageal adenocarcinoma incidence in the western world over the last two decades justifies the strong interest in BE and its development with the aim to improve preventative and therapeutic clinical strategies.

The histologic diagnosis of Barrett's dysplasia requires the identification of intestinal metaplasia, which often presents a challenge due to sampling error, observer variation, and difficulty in histologic interpretation. Particularly problematic is the separation of negative, indefinite, and low-grade dysplasia, the varied histological appearances of high-grade dysplasia, and the diagnosis of suboptimal biopsy material. This article seeks to aid in the histological evaluation of metaplasia and dysplasia in Barrett's esophagus.

This article reviews the epidemiology of Barrett's esophagus (BE) and current evidence for or against screening for BE to provide insight into the screening process. Data demonstrate that multiple criteria of a successful screening program remain unfulfilled or unproven in endoscopic screening for BE. The operating characteristics of the test are poorly described, and inadequate risk stratification limits the effectiveness and cost-effectiveness of the approach. We suggest modifications to BE screening practices that may have the potential to improve outcomes for patients with BE.

The incidence of esophageal adenocarcinoma (EAC) has increased dramatically in the western world, and there also appears to have been an increase in the incidence of Barrett's esophagus and gastroesophageal reflux disease in recent years. The contemporaneous increase in obesity has focused interest on whether obesity is a risk factor for EAC and its precursors. This article reviews current evidence for the role that overweight/obesity and body fat distribution have in development of the esophagitis metaplasia-dysplasia-adenocarcinoma sequence. Particular attention is paid to the stage at which adiposity may act to influence the risk of EAC, because this determines the importance of weight control and weight loss at each stage in the disease spectrum for the prevention of EAC.

This article focuses on the conceptual basis underlying the acquisition of each of the physiologic cancer hallmarks by metaplastic Barrett's cells. The acquired genetic alterations that have shown the most promise as potential molecular biomarkers to predict neoplastic progression in patients with Barrett's esophagus are reviewed. Moreover, the role of stem cells and stem cell markers in Barrett's carcinogenesis is addressed.

The incidence of esophageal adenocarcinoma is increasing at a rate greater than that of any other cancer in the Western world today. Barrett's esophagus is a clearly recognized risk factor for the development of esophageal adenocarcinoma, but the overwhelming majority of patients with Barrett's esophagus will never develop esophageal cancer. To date, dysplasia remains the only factor useful for identifying patients at increased risk for the development of esophageal adenocarcinoma in clinical practice. Other epidemiologic risk factors include aging, gender, race, obesity, reflux symptoms, smoking, and diet. Factors that may protect against the development of adenocarcinoma include infection with Helicobacter pylori, a diet rich in fruits and vegetables, and consumption of aspirin and NSAIDs.

There have been many developments in endoscopy-based imaging for the detection of Barrett's syndrome, dysplasia, and neoplasia in patients with Barrett's esophagus. This article reviews the studies on and compares the efficacy of several important endoscopic imaging modalities. Some of these technologies have already achieved regulatory approval, commercial availability, and establishment of clinical utility and practical application. The future of imaging for Barrett's syndrome likely rests with the development of molecular targeting with dysplasiatargeted probes that have been conjugated to dyes or nanoparticles.

The challenge of the title of this article is attention getting. How can medical therapy prevent cancer if anti-reflux surgery cannot prevent the neoplastic progression of Barrett's esophagus? Can anything short of esophagectomy prevent cancer? In the face of the increasing incidence of adenocarcinoma of the esophagus into the twenty-first century, the medical therapy of Barrett's esophagus and its potential role in preventing cancer are explored.

Endoscopic ablative therapy, and endoscopic mucosal resection (EMR) are the two general types of endoscopic therapies available for the treatment of Barrett's esophagus. The ablative therapies destroy metaplastic tissue, but do not provide a pathology specimen by which to judge the completeness of the ablation. In contrast, EMR provides large tissue specimens that can be examined by the pathologist to determine the character and extent of the mucosal abnormality and, for neoplastic lesions, the depth of involvement and the adequacy of resection. In this article, we discuss the use of endoscopic therapies for Barrett's esophagus presenting with no neoplasia, low and high-grade dysplasia, and early adenocarcinoma.

Patients diagnosed with Barrett's esophagus and high-grade dysplasia may harbor an intramucosal or early stage invasive esophageal carcinoma. The presence of and associated invasive malignancy exposes the patient to the risk of lymph node metastasis and its devastating effect on survival, regardless of treatment. The authors recommend that patients diagnosed with Barrett's esophagus and highgrade dysplasia be evaluated by an esophageal surgeon, who will be able to confirm the diagnosis and review the surgical options along with their potential benefits and risks. By continuously refining minimally invasive surgical techniques and perioperative care, esophageal resection should remain an acceptable option to patients with this disease.

This article examines the role of neoadjuvant therapy in the treatment of locally advanced esophageal adenocarcinoma. Recent studies have demonstrated that pre- or perioperative chemotherapy is associated with improved survival. Neoadjuvant chemoradiotherapy continues to be investigated but is associated with several advantages over neoadjuvant chemotherapy alone. Primary chemoradiotherapy is the accepted standard of care for medically inoperable patients, whereas adjuvant chemoradiotherapy may be considered for patients who undergo primary resection of lower esophageal/gastroesophageal junction tumors. Future directions include the investigation of newer chemotherapy regimens, the addition of targeted therapies, and the use of position emission tomography to provide an early assessment of response.

Adenocarcinoma arising in the setting of Barrett's esophagus has the fastest increasing incidence of any malignancy in the United States. Advanced esophageal cancer carries an overall poor prognosis with most patients presenting with incurable disease. Over the past several years, new options have been introduced for the purpose of providing palliative therapy to improve quality of life. Stent placement is the most widely used palliative therapy and rapidly relieves dysphagia; however, distal migration continues to be a disadvantage. Laser therapy and brachytherapy are also administered but require repeated treatment sessions. Future options for providing effective therapy for endstage disease include improved stent designs to decrease migration and multimodality methods that combine several options in one treatment session. This article focuses primarily on palliation of unresectable tumors of the esophagus and gastroesophageal junction.

RELATED INTEREST

Gastrointestinal Endoscopy Clinics of North America, July 2008 (Vol. 18, Number 3)
GI Cancer and the Endoscopist: Imaging and Treatment

THE CLINICS ARE NOW AVAILABLE ONLINE!

Access your subscription at:
www.theclinics.com

Foreword

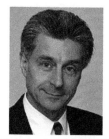

Nicholas J. Petrelli, MD
Consulting Editor

This issue of the *Surgical Oncology Clinics of North America* is devoted to Barrett's esophagus. The Guest Editor is Prateek Sharma, MD, Professor of Medicine and Director of the Gastrointestinal Fellowship Program at the University of Kansas School of Medicine.

Barrett's esophagus is an entity in which the composition of the cells lining the lower esophagus changes, not only in character but also in color because of repeated exposure to gastric acid, most often a result of long-term gastroesophageal reflux disease. The presence of Barrett's esophagus means there is a greater risk of developing esophageal cancer. Although increased, the absolute risk of esophageal cancer developing in an individual with Barrett's esophagus is less than 1% a year. Men are two to three times more likely to develop Barrett's esophagus than are women; and white and Hispanic people are at greater risk than are blacks and Asians. Although Barrett's esophagus can affect people of all ages, the condition is more common in older adults.

Dr. Sharma has put together an excellent edition of the *Surgical Oncology Clinics of North America*. This issue is a comprehensive review of Barrett's esophagus. Discussions center around the cellular mechanisms, the histology of metaplasia and dysplasia, and the improvement of screening practices. Other interesting discussions center around the risk factors and new technologies for imaging, along with the role of neoadjuvant therapy for Barrett's esophageal cancer. The authors contributing to this issue are experts in this field and have been chosen by Dr. Sharma because of their experience.

As Dr. Sharma states in the preface, "This issue should provide clinicians with better knowledge about the various approaches to treatment of patients with Barrett's esophagus and esophageal cancer." I have read these articles and totally agree with

Surg Oncol Clin N Am 18 (2009) xiii–xiv
doi:10.1016/j.soc.2009.04.002
surgonc.theclinics.com

Dr. Sharma. I encourage attending staff to share this issue with their medical students, residents, and fellows in training.

Nicholas J. Petrelli, MD
Helen F. Graham Cancer Center
Christiana Care Health System
4701 Ogletown-Stanton Road
Suite 1233
Newark, DE19713
Department of Surgery
Thomas Jefferson University
1021 Walnut Street
Philadelphia, PA 19107

E-mail address:
npetrelli@christianacare.org (N.J. Petrelli)

Preface

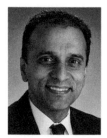

Prateek Sharma, MD
Guest Editor

The rise in the incidence of esophageal adenocarcinoma has been witnessed in the United States and in the entire western world. Mortality rates from this cancer have paralleled this increase in incidence. Barrett's esophagus, as a premalignant lesion, is recognized in the majority of cases of adenocarcinoma of the esophagus and esophagogastric junction. Increasing attention has been focused on the diagnosis and detection of early neoplasia in Barrett's esophagus. This focus has improved our understanding of the possible causes leading to the rise in cancer incidence. It also has fostered the use of minimally invasive therapies including endoscopic therapy.

Endoscopy with biopsy is currently the only standardized and validated technique to diagnose Barrett's esophagus. However, the use of techniques such as high-definition endoscopy, chromoendoscopy with or without magnification, and endoscopic optical techniques such as narrow-band imaging and confocal microscopy may allow us to obtain us "real time" biopsies of the esophagus. Cost-effectiveness of surveillance in patients with Barrett's esophagus is connected to the incidence of adenocarcinoma. Accurate risk stratification of patients (ie, identifying those at the highest risk for cancer) would reduce the number of patients requiring surveillance and our limited health care resources could then be focused on the high-risk group. Risk stratification and improvements to our methods for diagnosis of dysplasia and cancer could be enhanced—leading to significant improvements in screening and surveillance of Barrett's esophagus. Thus, the goal is the use of an effective tool to detect Barrett's esophagus, dysplasia, or cancer in high-risk populations at the lowest cost and at minimum risk. Finally, endoscopic techniques and minimally invasive esophagectomy can probably play a role for patients with high-grade dysplasia or early adenocarcinoma.

In this issue, experts in the field of Barrett's esophagus and esophageal cancer discuss the causes, epidemiology, endoscopic diagnosis, use of endoscopic techniques, and the role of medical and surgical interventions. All the authors have provided in-depth reviews of their topic with extremely useful clinical information. This issue should provide clinicians with better knowledge about the various approaches to treatment of patients with Barrett's esophagus and esophageal cancer.

Surg Oncol Clin N Am 18 (2009) xv–xvi
doi:10.1016/j.soc.2009.04.003
1055-3207/09/$ – see front matter © 2009 Elsevier Inc. All rights reserved.

surgonc.theclinics.com

I want to thank all the authors for uniformly providing detailed and practical reviews of their topics, and Mary Mackison and Catherine Bewick for their help with the preparation of this issue.

Prateek Sharma, MD
Professor of Medicine
Director of Gastrointestinal Fellowship Program
University of Kansas School of Medicine
VA Medical Center
Kansas City, MO

E-mail address:
psharma@kumc.edu (P. Sharma)

Cellular Mechanisms of Barrett's Esophagus Development

Mariagnese Barbera, PhD[a],
Rebecca C. Fitzgerald, MA (Cantab), MD, FRCP[b,c,d],*

KEYWORDS

• Metaplasia • Stem cells • GERD • Acid • Bile

Barrett's esophagus (BE) is a metaplastic premalignant disorder in which the normal stratified squamous epithelium of the lower esophagus is replaced by a columnar lined epithelium with intestinal differentiation. BE generally occurs in the context of chronic gastroesophageal reflux disease (GERD), and it is the primary risk factor for the development of esophageal adenocarcinoma with a conversion rate of 0.5% to 1% per annum. The dramatic increase of esophageal adenocarcinoma incidence in the western world over the last two decades justifies the strong interest in BE and its development with the aim to improve preventative and therapeutic clinical strategies.

METAPLASIA AND ORIGIN OF BARRETT'S EPITHELIUM

Metaplasia is the process whereby, during postnatal life, there is general transformation of one tissue type into another. Metaplasia is commonly associated with increased cell proliferation and may progress to dysplasia and, eventually, cancer. BE is a classic example of metaplasia. In general, metaplasia can arise from wound healing, prolonged tissue stress, or in response to abnormal tissue stimulation.[1] The importance of the luminal environment, and in particular reflux components, as a trigger for BE has been widely established.[2] The cellular and molecular mechanisms involved in BE development are still poorly understood, however, and this is at least in part caused by the difficulties in observing this process *in vivo* and the lack of reliable animal models. The origin of BE is still controversial, and several hypotheses have been proposed to define and identify the cells that give rise to the metaplastic tissue.

[a] Hutchison-MRC Research Centre, Hills Road, Cambridge, CB2 0XZ, UK
[b] MRC Cancer Cell Unit, Hutchison-MRC Research Centre, Hills Road, Cambridge, CB2 0XZ, UK
[c] Department of Gastroenterology, Addenbrooke's Hospital, Cambridge, UK
[d] Department of General Mediciane, Addenbrooke's Hospital, Cambridge, UK
* Corresponding author. MRC Cancer Cell Unit, Hutchison-MRC Research Centre, Hills Road, Cambridge, CB2 0XZ, UK.
E-mail address: rcf@hutchison-mrc.cam.ac.uk (R.C. Fitzgerald).

Surg Oncol Clin N Am 18 (2009) 393–410
doi:10.1016/j.soc.2009.03.001
surgonc.theclinics.com
1055-3207/09/$ – see front matter © 2009 Elsevier Inc. All rights reserved.

Initially, BE was thought to arise as a consequence of upward cell migration from the transitional zone cells of the gastroesophageal junction[3] and it was proposed that these cells migrate and colonize the distal esophagus or the gastric cardia in response to tissue damage from continued toxic exposure to refluxate (**Fig. 1**A). Recently, a study on the distribution of esophageal and gastric cardiac mucosae in esophagectomy specimens led to the suggestion that cardiac glands are exposed to the luminal surface and become columnar epithelial islands, which could clonally expand to give rise to BE.[4] Nevertheless, in animal models, columnar epithelium can still develop in defective mucosa above a squamous barrier, which separates the distal esophagus from the transitional zone of the stomach.[5] Furthermore, even if damage from refluxate can lead to gastric cell migration, one still needs to account for the different epithelial cell lineages in BE.

The second hypothesis assigns the origin of BE to a subclass of metaplasia called "transdifferentiation" (**Fig. 1**B). This term describes an irreversible metaplastic conversion from one fully differentiated state to another.[1] A study of the conversion of the epithelium from columnar to stratified squamous during the development of the embryonic esophagus in the mouse supports this hypothesis.[6] It was shown that a proportion of cells coexpress markers of squamous (cytokeratin 14) and columnar (cytokeratin 8) differentiation during the columnar-squamous conversion.[6] The authors suggest that squamous esophageal cells can arise directly from columnar basal cells, independent of cell division or apoptosis. The reverse transformation could account for the switch in phenotype in BE. Whether this switch can occur in adulthood, however, remains to be proved. Furthermore, evidence of new squamous epithelium that develops after the endoscopic removal of Barrett's epithelium[7] (assuming that the differentiated epithelium was completely removed) weakens the theory of transdifferentiation. A related hypothesis suggests a role for an intermediate multilayered epithelium that expresses cytokeratins of both squamous and columnar differentiation. This is composed of multiple layers of cells that appear squamous in their basal portion and columnar more superficially.[8]

Another possibility is that Barrett's metaplasia results from a change in the commitment of multipotent stem cells, which are led to differentiate into columnar rather than squamous epithelium, as a result of the continuous exposure to environmental stresses, such as refluxate. The stem cells of the esophageal epithelium are believed to reside in the interpapillary basal layer (**Fig. 1**C).[9] According to this model, slowly dividing stem cells in the basal layer generate transit amplifying cells, which reside in the epibasal layer and maintain the stem cell compartment. On commitment to terminal differentiation, transit amplifying cells undergo a few rounds of division and, eventually, their progeny differentiate into squamous keratinocytes. The current model of homeostasis in esophageal epithelium, however, is still an active area of research. With the advent of new molecular techniques it is now possible to study the fate of the progeny of an individual stem cell using *in vivo* lineage tracing. A recent study performed on mouse tail skin, using inducible genetic labeling, demonstrated that the clone-size distributions were consistent with a new model of homeostasis.[10] This model involves one single type of progenitor cell that divides stochastically with a certain fixed ratio, generating three possible combinations of cell progeny: (1) two undifferentiated progenitor cells, (2) two cells committed to differentiation, or (3) one undifferentiated progenitor cell and one committed to differentiation. These results raise important questions about the potential role of stem cells, which would not participate in the normal homeostasis of the epithelium but would only intervene in the case of tissue damage. Similar lines of enquiry in the esophagus may be informative.

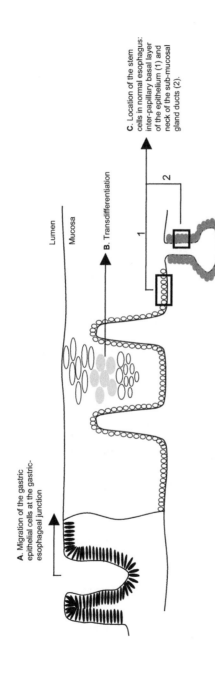

Fig. 1. Theories for the cell origin of Barrett's metaplasia. (A) Epithelial cells at the gastroesophageal junction migrate and colonize the distal esophagus. (B) Transdifferentiation, the irreversible switch of the phenotype of adult differentiated epithelial cells. (C) Stem cells of the normal esophagus, after chronic exposure to refluxate, are reprogrammed to differentiate in a columnar phenotype, rather than squamous. Stem cells in the epithelium of normal esophagus are thought to be located in the basal layer of the epithelium (1) and in the neck of the esophageal submucosal gland ducts (2).

A second population of stem cells may be located in the glandular neck region of the esophageal submucosal gland ducts, similar to those found in the bulge region of the hair follicles (see **Fig. 1C**).[11] Because ducts are lined in their proximal two thirds by columnar cells, whereas their distal third is lined with squamous cells,[12] this stem cell population has been proposed as a possible source for the columnar epithelium. This hypothesis is based on the ulcer-associated cell lineage[13] that occurs adjacent to areas of ulceration in the gastrointestinal tract, and prefigures a migration of the glandular cells to the surface, through new glands and ducts generated by stem cells in the lamina propria.[14] The gland duct theory has recently been the subject of several studies that seem to support the concept that these calls may be critical for the development of BE. A study using retinoic acid as a stimulus for cell differentiation suggested that the stromal compartment, which includes the submucosal gland ducts, is the cell source for the columnar cells induced by retinoic acid treatment of squamous tissue.[15] An immunohistochemical characterization study in pig tissues and cultures indicated similarities between the submucosal glands and BE.[16] A histologic study on serial sections of esophageal resection tissue showed frequent gland ducts opening onto the surface of Barrett's epithelium.[14] A study on individual epithelial crypts has recently demonstrated that Barrett's heterogeneity arises from multiple independent clones. Furthermore, a p16 mutation in common between the submucosal gland duct and adjacent Barrett's epithelium was found, suggesting a common genetic origin for these cells.[17] In a similar study islands of neosquamous epithelium were found to be wild-type at loci containing mutations within the adjacent Barrett's epithelium. This suggests that the neosquamous epithelium originates in different cells from those responsible for self-renewal of the Barrett's epithelium and gland ducts are a possible source.[18] Finally, it has been suggested that BE could originate from bone marrow–derived stem cells,[19] and although currently there are little data on this in the context of BE, similar evidence has been found in gastric intestinal metaplasia.[20]

The idea that reprogramming of stem cells plays a causal role in the pathogenesis of BE is relatively new and interesting. It has been reported that duodenal juice stimulates esophageal stem cells to induce BE in rats.[21] More recently, with immunohistochemical and quantitative polymerase chain reaction techniques in the human gastric epithelium, it has been demonstrated that multiple mutated multipotent stem cells can colonize the entire unit, resulting in a new clonal unit by a process called "monoclonal conversion."[22] The authors of the study proposed that monoclonal conversion could be a mechanism for the colonization of gastric crypts seen in intestinal metaplasia, whereby gastric stem cells commit to the intestinal phenotype. The stem cell theory could also explain how a variety of phenotypes are observed characterizing the cell population in BE, and the development of new squamous epithelium after complete removal of BE.

Further research is required to understand the development of the Barrett's epithelium bearing in mind that it may originate from more than one source.

ROLE OF GASTROESOPHAGEAL REFLUX DISEASE AND ACID EXPOSURE

It has been clearly established that GERD is the main risk factor for the development of BE.[2] GERD typically causes heartburn symptoms and can lead to a spectrum of abnormalities of the esophageal mucosa including esophagitis, strictures, discrete ulcers, and BE. The composition of refluxate may vary between individuals but normally includes oroesophageal, gastric, and duodenal contents. The extent to which the specific components of the refluxate contributes to the disease pathogenesis is not fully elucidated but there are data to support a role for acid and bile.

It has been hypothesized that BE develops as a defense mechanism in response to repeated exposure to low pH over a prolonged period. The mechanisms are thought to include chronic inflammation, oxidative stress, and mitochondrial and DNA damage before leading to a columnar metaplasia.[2] In the early 1970s, an experiment was conducted in which removal of the distal esophageal mucosa was followed by repeated injections of histamine to induce acid secretion. This resulted in the development of a columnar mucosa demonstrating that acid reflux injury is necessary for the development of BE.[23] Later, it was demonstrated that BE patients have an increased exposure to acid refluxate compared with those with erosive esophagitis and nonerosive reflux disesase.[24] Furthermore, in a clinical 24-hour esophageal pH study a significant relationship was observed between the rate of change in acid exposure and the length of Barrett's mucosa.[25] Numerous studies have investigated the therapeutic effectiveness of intraesophageal acid suppression in the regression of BE and the prevention of cancer development. The elimination of acid reflux results in partial regression of the Barrett's segment.[26] Using surrogate indicators of cancer risk investigators have shown that effective normalization of intraesophageal pH in BE patients favors differentiation and decreased proliferation of the epithelium.[27] Recently, a large retrospective clinical study demonstrated that the use of proton pumps inhibitors before a diagnosis of BE remarkably reduces the risk of high-grade dysplasia.[28] Although these data suggest that acid suppression may prevent cancer progression, caution has to be exercised in interpreting these surrogate markers. Overall, the implications for the risk of cancer development are still not completely clear and a direct relationship between acid-suppression therapy and prevention of malignant progression has not yet been established. For example, it has been showed that by comparing complete and incomplete acid suppression with the expression of proliferation, apoptosis, and inflammatory markers in BE patients, long-term acid suppression reduces proliferation, but has no significant effect on apoptosis or expression of cyclooxygenase-2 (COX2),[29] nor does it reduce the formation of DNA adducts caused by oxidative damage.[30]

The mechanism of acid injury depends on the ability of H^+ ions to cross the epithelial cell membrane, enter the cytoplasm, and significantly decrease the intracellular pH (**Fig. 2A**). Because of the low permeability of the apical membrane to acid, the luminal pH has to be low enough to damage the intercellular junction structures, and increase the intercellular space, to allow H^+ ions to penetrate through the basolateral membrane. The transporters could be the same as those used in the regulation of intracellular pH, such as the Na independent Cl/HCO_3 exchanger.[31] Recently, a physiologic and molecular analysis of acid-loading mechanisms demonstrated qualitative and quantitative differences in the acid loading between columnar and squamous esophageal cells.[32] Barrett's cells use an additional Na/H^+ ion exchange mechanism for acid loading in addition to the Na independent Cl/HCO_3 exchange used by squamous epithelial cells. In these conditions, H^+ ions cause cell necrosis, which results in ulceration of the tissue when the damage extends over a large area. BE cells, however, seem to withstand repeated acid injury better than their squamous counterparts.

The molecular events leading to necrosis are still not completely understood, but it has been proposed that the low pH could inhibit K^+ channels[33] and as a consequence cells lose the capability to regulate their volume. Another hypothesis is that the inhibition of the Na/K ATPase pump induces a progressive and irreversible decrease in the membrane electric potential, which leads to cell death.[34]

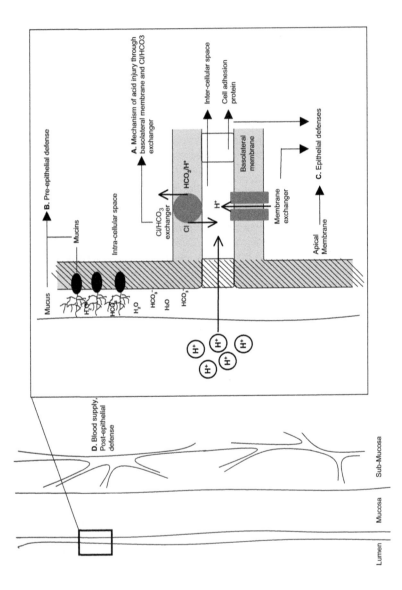

Fig. 2. Acid injury to the esophageal epithelium and mechanisms of defense. (A) H+ ions from the esophageal lumen penetrate inside the cell, by passing through the membrane. Because of the low permeability of the apical membrane the luminal pH has to be low enough to damage the inter-cellular junction structures and allow H+ ions to reach the basolateral membrane through which they are transported by Na-independent Cl/HCO3 exchanger. (B) The esophagus has three different mechanisms of defense to acid damage. The pre-epithelial defense comes from the mucus-unstirred water and bicarbonate layer complex, which is mainly glycol-conjugate with mucins. (C) The epithelial defense is constituted by the apical membrane barrier including cell-cell adhesion proteins and membrane exchangers. (D) The postepithelial defense comes from the vascular network.

Epithelial Defense Mechanisms

The mechanisms of defense used by the esophageal epithelium against acid can be divided into pre-epithelial, epithelial, and postepithelial. The pre-epithelial defenses (**Fig. 2**B) include the mucus-unstirred water and bicarbonate layer complex, which is mainly glycol-conjugate with mucins. Both qualitative and quantitative changes in glycol-conjugate secretion have been observed in BE such that the rate of glycol-conjugate release is changed significantly according to the endoluminal pH,[35] and the pattern of mucin gene expression is modified compared with squamous epithelium.[36] In particular, expression of mucins that correlate with gastric differentiation (MUC5AC and MUC6) and with intestinal differentiation (MUC2) has been identified. The epithelial defenses (**Fig. 2**C) are mainly conferred by the cell membrane barrier and, in particular, by the membrane exchangers, whose activity could be significantly damaged by an overexposure to acid.[37] An adequate blood supply constitutes the major postepithelial defense (**Fig. 2**D), and a remarkable increase of the blood flow in the lower esophagus has been demonstrated in consequence to an acidic luminal environment.[38] Further work is required to understand fully the molecular pathways triggered by acid exposure in the development of BE.

Role of Duodenal Contents

In addition to acid there is also evidence for a role of duodenal juice in the development of BE, which may explain why BE can develop in patients who have undergone total gastrectomy[39] and esophagectomy.[40] Furthermore, BE has been reported in a rat model in which the esophagus is joined to the duodenum and not exposed to acid refluxate.[41] The effects of this surgery seems to be species dependent, however, because in rabbits these components induced severe esophagitis.[42] More recent studies have focused on the relationship between duodenal juice and CDX2, a transcription factor involved in the differentiation and maintenance of intestinal epithelium that is overexpressed in BE.[43] CDX2 belongs to the family of homeobox, genes that are developmental transcription factors responsible for body patterning during embryogenesis. These genes are expressed, along the length of the gut, according to the location of the gene in the chromosome. CDX2 is characterized by a caudal distribution, being mainly expressed in the small intestine and colon but not in the stomach or in the esophagus. In both rats exposed to duodenal refluxate[44] and human cells treated with primary and secondary bile acids[45] up-regulation of CDX2 was detected. Furthermore, it has been demonstrated that bile acids directly increase the production of CDX2 in rat esophageal keratinocytes, with expression of intestinal-type mucin.[46]

Role of Chronic Inflammation

In addition to the direct cytotoxic effect of H^+ ions, the main consequence of a prolonged and sustained acid and bile acid exposure is a chronic inflammatory response, which in turn causes epithelial damage. Inflammation is associated with production of free-radicals and reactive oxygen species, which leads to depletion of antioxidants, oxidative stress, and increased expression of genes involved in the regulation of the redox balance, such as thioredoxin reductase.[47] Up-regulation of enzymes, such as nitric oxide synthase, COX2, and myeloperoxidase, has been identified during the development of BE and also in the progression to cancer.[48] The induction of inducible nitric oxide synthase is not the only possible source of nitric oxide radical. Dietary nitrates have been shown to be a source of luminal nitric oxide[49] and an *in vitro* and *ex vivo* study demonstrated that luminal nitric oxide secondary to dietary nitrate is able to induce double-strand DNA breaks.[50] Increased COX2 activity results in activation of the biosynthetic pathway of prostaglandins, which may be relevant for the inflammatory induction of metaplasia. An *in vivo* study that investigated the changes in the expression of COX1, COX2, and microsomial prostaglandin E synthase-1 in a rat model of duodenal reflux showed that microsomial prostaglandin E synthase-1 was highly expressed in stromal tissue and corresponded with COX2 expression.[51] Furthermore, the ability of acid and bile salts to induce oxidative DNA damage *in vitro* was demonstrated in two esophageal cell lines.[52] Recently, a study on hTERT immortalized squamous cell lines derived from GERD patients with and without BE and a BE cell line, demonstrated that both NADPH oxidase and nitric oxide synthase contributed to the production of reactive oxygen species in squamous cells from GERD patients without BE, whereas only NADPH oxidase is responsible for the generation of reactive oxygen species in cells from BE patients.[53] The authors proposed that the different mechanisms of reflux-induced oxidant production could play a significant role in the determination of disease progression.

Role of Immune Factors

In addition to toxic oxygen species, immune factors are also recruited as part of the inflammatory response and may be relevant to the origin of BE. An immunohistochemical study of samples from BE patients showed that the IL-6/STAT3 antiapoptotic pathway is induced by exposure to bile acid and low pH.[54] Another study performed through immunohistochemical and Western blot analysis of BE samples demonstrated that levels of tumor necrosis factor-α are increased in BE tissue compared with normal epithelium.[55] Evidence from the same study showed that the tumor necrosis factor-α expression increased in the progression toward cancer. An immunohistochemical quantitative analysis of Th1 and Th2 effector cells in biopsies from BE and reflux esophagitis patients was performed to detect the antibody classes produced by plasma cells and to determine the presence of isolated lymph follicles.[56] The results demonstrated that BE samples expressed a higher proportion of Th2 effectors, levels of IgE+ plasma cells, and frequency of isolated lymph follicles compared with esophagitis samples. The authors suggested that BE is characterized by a Th2 response in keeping with two previous studies that investigated the interleukin expression profile in long-segment BE[57] and in BE compared with esophagitis and nonerosive reflux disease.[58] In BE, although a Th2 cytokine profile predominated in the distal segment, a proinflammatory response was seen in the esophagitis-associated squamocolumnar junction in BE. The type of immune response generated may be important in the ability of the host to evade invasion by the tumor[59] and this may be genetically predetermined. For example, a genetic profile predisposing to a strong proinflammatory host response, mediated by IL-12p20 and partially dependent on IL-10, has been demonstrated in patients with BE compared with those with reflux esophagitis.[60] Very large sample sizes are needed, however, to substantiate these findings. This is now becoming feasible through the large population-based cohort studies and the technologic advances in single nucleotide polymorphism genotyping.

With regards to the clinical applicability of these findings, although a number of issues concerning the role of reflux exposure and the inflammatory response are still under investigation, there is an increasing body of evidence to demonstrate that the high levels of acid and bile within the esophageal lumen, in association with specific inflammatory responses, are linked to the pathogenesis of BE. For this reason acid suppression and control of GERD is still an important therapeutic strategy for the treatment of BE, although data from prospective randomized controlled trials are required to confirm the cancer preventive efficacy of this approach.

DEVELOPMENT OF GENETIC ALTERATIONS AND THEIR ROLE IN BARRETT'S ESOPHAGUS

The pathogenesis of BE is associated with the establishment of several genetic and epigenetic alterations, which represent the first step in a series of events that may result in the development of adenocarcinoma. None of these somatic alterations has been identified as pivotal, but their combination and accumulation enable cells to express a Barrett's metaplastic phenotype with the capacity for malignant progression.

At the chromosomal level, BE is characterized by genetic instability that results in gene rearrangements, aneuploidy,[61] allelic imbalance,[62] and possibly microsatellite instability.[63] Measurement of DNA content in samples from BE patients has shown increased aneuploidy levels in metaplastic tissue, compared with adjacent normal esophageal and gastric epithelium.[64] Aneuploidy has also been identified as an important event in the evolution of metaplasia to adenocarcinoma,[65] and it has been proposed as a possible biomarker for cancer risk stratification in BE.[66] A thorough chromosomal analysis showed that allelic imbalance is a frequent event in BE and is independent of the gastric or intestinal phenotype.[62] Interestingly, instability in the DNA sequence has also been detected in microsatellites, even before the onset of aneuploidy.[63] Microsatellites are repeating units of small DNA sequences that vary in length and are uniformly spread throughout the genome. Microsatellite instability occurs when rapid cell proliferation causes mismatch repair of genes and modification of the microsatellite sequence size. The degree of microsatellite instability in BE is frequently small,[67] however, and the mismatch repair genes involved have not yet been clearly identified; the actual contribution of this event in the pathogenesis of BE is still under investigation.

Generalized DNA damage is another frequently observed event in BE. DNA analysis of BE biopsies has been performed by comparing columnar and squamous epithelium from the same BE patients,[68] or by evaluating columnar, squamous, and gastric epithelium samples from BE patients using squamous biopsies from healthy patients as a control.[69] In both cases, remarkably higher levels of DNA damage were identified in the metaplastic samples, compared with the reference samples. The most frequent types of damage detected included strand breaks, alkali-labile sites, and ring-opened purine lesions. The nature of the damage observed is consistent with the presence of free radical species, as a consequence of oxidative stress, caused by the exposure to an acidic environment.[52]

Besides nonspecific damage, specific gene modifications are also an important cause of the most typical functional abnormalities in BE cell. Most of these features, which include switches in the differentiation status and increased-uncoordinated proliferation related to alteration of the cell cycle control, are strongly involved also in the development of dysplasia and cancer. The malignant progression is beyond the scope of this article, however, and only the genetic abnormalities that occur early in the metaplasia-dysplasia-carcinoma sequence are discussed.

In metaplastic transformation of esophageal epithelium from squamous to columnar, genetic alterations of determinants of cell fate and differentiation are necessary. One theory that could explain the mechanism of cell fate deregulation involves an abnormal switch of genes involved in the physiologic transition from columnar to squamous in embryogenesis in response to an external injury.[70] Injury could cause perturbations in the transcription status of genes in an adult squamous multipotent stem cell, and lead either to inactivation of genes essential for the expression of squamous phenotype, or reactivation of genes related with the development of columnar features.[1]

p63, a member of the p53 family, which regulates differentiation and morphogenesis in epithelial tissue, is required for the formation of the squamous epithelia, and is normally absent in columnar epithelium. The critical and essential role of p63 in the development of a normal esophageal epithelium has been demonstrated in a model of p63$^{(-/-)}$ mice that developed a columnar ciliated esophageal epithelium.[71] In samples with varying degrees of dysplasia and neoplasia from patients who underwent esophageal resection, despite high levels of p63 gene expression, very low expression levels of the protein were detectable.[72] Interestingly, down-regulation of p63 after exposure of a normal esophageal cell line to bile salt and acid has been observed.[73]

CDX2 is another candidate gene for the differentiation switch in BE. In keeping with this the activity of CDX2 has been related to the transcription of genes strictly involved in the intestinal differentiation, such as MUC2.[74] Overexpression of CDX2 in BE and intestinal metaplasia of the stomach has been clearly demonstrated in humans.[43] CDX2 has also been proposed as a possible biomarker to detect early transition from squamous mucosa to BE.[75] Presence of CDX2 mRNA has been observed in squamous biopsies of BE patients, suggesting that a switch in phenotype might follow the abnormal expression of the protein.[76] Studies on transgenic mice expressing ectopic CDX2 in the stomach showed that the animal developed intestinal metaplasia, confirmed by the expression of specific intestinal genes, such as villin and MUC2.[77] Recently, both *in vitro* and *in vivo* studies linked the overexpression of CDX2 with the abnormal exposure to bile acid and salts.

It has been suggested that abnormalities in the G1-S phase progression are mainly responsible for the deregulation of the cell cycle control at the early stage of the disease.[78] The significance of this is unclear, however, when one takes into account the overall increase in cell number during the metaplasia-dysplasia-carcinoma sequence.[79] Cyclin D1, a known oncogene, plays a key role in the regulation of cell cycle progression from G1 to S phase and its main function involves the coordination of mitogenic and differentiation signaling pathways. Aberrant cyclin D1 expression has been related to genetic instability *in vitro* and tumorigenesis *in vivo*. In an immunohistochemical study that investigated the levels of cyclin D1 in BE surveillance biopsies, nuclear overexpression of the protein has been observed in up to 46% of the samples, as compared with normal squamous epithelium.[80] Cyclin D1 is also characterized by adenine-guanine single nucleotide polymorphism in exon 4, which is associated with two different splice-variant transcripts. The variant leading to a shorter cyclin D1 protein with a longer half-life has been shown to have oncogenic properties.[81] Cyclin E acts by binding to G_1 phase CDK2 and it is essential for the transition from G_1 to S phase. Increased expression of this protein has been observed in paraffin-embedded BE biopsies compared with normal adjacent mucosa.[82] Increasing levels of cyclin A were also detected in a study that performed a comprehensive analysis of the overall proliferation status and cell cycle stage distribution in BE-associated using immunohistochemistry and flow cytometry.[79] Following on from this a clinical study suggested that cyclin A might be useful as a risk stratification tool for BE surveillance.[83]

Uncontrolled cell growth can also be caused by a severe imbalance of proliferation and apoptosis, which involves the aberrant expression of tumor suppressor genes, among which the most significant is p53. Although alterations of p53 have been mainly related to the neoplastic progression, p53 mutations have also been reported in the early phase of BE, with a rate that varies from 50% to 90%,[84] and loss of heterozygosity of p53 (17p allelic loss) has been detected in the nonmalignant stage of the disease.[85] Furthermore, immunohistochemical studies have confirmed molecular alterations of TP53 in BE without dysplasia[86] and its overexpression indicates the presence of a mutated form that has a longer half-life than the wild-type.[87] In BE, loss of p53 might have particular implication in aneuploidy. A study of the relationship between p53 loss of heterozygosity, abnormal cell cycle fractions, and aneuploidy in BE showed that identical p53 mutations are expressed in both diploid and aneuploidy populations.[88] These results suggest that aneuploidy occurs after p53 mutation, possibly as a consequence of the abnormal cycling. p53 is involved in a number of network pathways and its activity is related to many other factors that act indirectly affecting the expression of the tumor suppressor. Among them is p14ARF, a key regulator of the p53 tumor suppressor pathway, which seems to be silenced progressively by epigenetic mechanisms in the progression to adenocarcinoma.[89]

Mutations in p16 represent another critical factor implicated in the deregulation of cell cycle and proliferation, which occurs in BE. p16 gene is located on chromosome 9, acts as upstream regulator of p53 pathways, and controls progression of cell cycle at the G1/S checkpoint by binding and deactivating various cyclin-cyclin–dependent kinase complexes. The p16 gene locus is well known for very frequent homozygous and heterozygous deletions, point mutations, and epigenetic changes, which result in p16 inactivation and are a typical feature in tumorigenesis. Significant evidence links alteration of p16 function with the early stage of BE and, consequently, of esophageal adenocarcinoma. Allelic loss of 9p21 locus and mutation of p16 gene were detected in populations of aneuploid cells from premalignant BE.[90] A DNA sequencing study showed that in biopsies from BE patients, 57% of the samples were characterized by loss of heterozygosity for p16 and more than 85% of Barrett's segment had clones with one or two p16 lesions.[91] The authors also found that the p16 deletion status related to an increase in the length of Barrett's segment. In a following study the status of p16 expression and methylation was examined and the results confirmed that inactivation of p16 occurs already in BE and suggested that the main cause of inactivation of its locus is a promoter methylation. A robust study has been performed using biopsies from BE patients to evaluate the expansion of genetic lesions in Barrett's segments by measuring the proportion of proliferating cells that carried those particular lesions.[92] The results showed that p16 heterozygosity, promoter methylation, and sequence mutations have strong, independent, and advantageous effects on BE onset. Mutations of p16 would act as selective "hitchhikers" and contribute to clonal expansion and disease progression.[93]

The uncontrolled cell proliferation, typical of BE, could also be a result of derangement in the normal cell senescence process leading to immortalization of the metaplastic epithelial cell population. The main mechanism of cell senescence involves shortening of telomeres. In BE, increase in RNA expression of telomerase, the enzyme that prevents cell senescence by maintaining constant the length of telomeres, has been reported in biopsies from BE patients and surgical resection specimens of esophageal adenocarcinoma containing varying stages of neoplastic progression.[94] A subsequent study that investigated mRNA expression levels of telomerase reverse-transcriptase catalytic subunit (hTERT) demonstrated that its expression was significantly increased at all stages of BE, suggesting that telomerase activation is an important early event in the development of the disease.[95]

In addition to typical genetic modifications caused by sequence alterations, metaplastic epithelium is also characterized by epigenetic alterations (methylation and histone modifications) and post-transcriptional non–sequence-based events that are inherited through cell division and play a pivotal role in the regulation of gene expression. One key example is p16, as mentioned previously. Promoter hypermethylation was one of the first epigenetic events identified as a common mechanism of p16 gene inactivation in the development of BE.[96] More recently, p16 promoter hypermethylation has been detected in 77% of surgically resected esophageal tissues from BE patients.[97] Furthermore, DNA analysis for inactivation of the locus of p16 in BE samples showed that methylation of p16 seems to be the most frequent epigenetic defect in BE and in its progression to cancer.[98] More recently, particular interest has risen toward the adenomatous polyposis coli, a gene that connects cadherins with actin filaments and acts as a tumor suppressor gene through its regulatory role in the Wnt/βcatenin signaling pathway. Epigenetic silencing of the Wnt inhibitory factor–1, through promoter methylation, has been demonstrated as a common event that precedes BE carcinogenesis.[99] Hypermethylation of the adenomatous polyposis coli promoter has been observed in 92% of patients with esophageal adenocarcinoma and could be detected in BE precursor lesions.[100] In a study that investigated the expression pattern of several proteins involved in the Wnt signaling pathway complete methylation of adenomatous polyposis coli, which correlated with lack of expression, was found in 100% of the BE samples.[101] Another likely target for epigenetic regulation is CDX2. Although a specific study has not been performed yet on BE, down-regulation of CDX2 by DNA methylation has been shown in several cell populations, such as embryonic stem cells and in colon cancer.[102] Using Het-1A cells, an immortalized cell line of normal squamous esophagus, CDX2 expression was repressed by DNA methylation and then reactivated through the treatment with 5-aza-2'deoxycytidine.[103] Other genes that undergo promoter hypermethylation and following silencing in BE are nel-like 1,[104] located on cromosome11p15, which frequently undergoes loss of heterozygosity in esophageal adenocarcinoma, and AKAP12,[105] a kinase scaffold protein with known tumor suppressor activity. Understanding of epigenetic events in BE is still in its infancy.

Overall, the genetic and epigenetic modifications underlying the development of BE represent a very complex process involving numerous factors whose role is still not completely clear. Barrett's metaplastic cells are characterized by a particular susceptibility to DNA damage that, coupled with inflammatory response to bile salts and acid exposure, may trigger further genetic alterations that undergo clonal selection and expansion and promote progression to cancer.

SUMMARY

It is reasonable to hypothesize that the development of BE is the result of changes in the microenvironment of one or more cell populations within the squamous esophageal tissue, which might be either multipotent progenitor cells or adult differentiated cells. Chronic exposure to the gastric and bile reflux components of that microenvironment may lead to fundamental alterations in the transcriptional programming of these cells, altering their cell fate determination to an intestinal lineage. Continued tissue damage leads to nonspecific DNA damage and an accumulation of genetic and epigenetic alterations, which drives clones with a selective advantage to become dominant with the potential for cancer development.

REFERENCES

1. Tosh D, Slack JM. How cells change their phenotype. Nat Rev Mol Cell Biol 2002; 3:187–94.
2. Vaezi MF, Richter JE. Role of acid and duodenogastroesophageal reflux in gastroesophageal reflux disease. Gastroenterology 1996;111:1192–9.

3. Hamilton SR, Yardley JH. Regnerative of cardiac type mucosa and acquisition of Barrett mucosa after esophagogastrostomy. Gastroenterology 1977;72: 669–75.

4. Nakanishi Y, Saka M, Eguchi T, et al. Distribution and significance of the oeso-phageal and gastric cardiac mucosae: a study of 131 operation specimens. Histopathology 2007;51:515–9.

5. Li H, Walsh TN, O'Dowd G, et al. Mechanisms of columnar metaplasia and squa-mous regeneration in experimental Barrett's esophagus. Surgery 1994;115: 176–81.

6. Yu WY, Slack JM, Tosh D. Conversion of columnar to stratified squamous epithe-lium in the developing mouse oesophagus. Dev Biol 2005;284:157–70.

7. Barham CP, Jones RL, Biddlestone LR, et al. Photothermal laser ablation of Bar-rett's oesophagus: endoscopic and histological evidence of squamous re-epi-thelialisation. Gut 1997;41:281–4.

8. Shields HM, Rosenberg SJ, Zwas FR, et al. Prospective evaluation of multilay-ered epithelium in Barrett's esophagus. Am J Gastroenterol 2001;96:3268–73.

9. Seery JP. Stem cells of the oesophageal epithelium. J Cell Sci 2002;115:1783–9.

10. Clayton E, Doupe DP, Klein AM, et al. A single type of progenitor cell maintains normal epidermis. Nature 2007;446:185–9.

11. Rochat A, Kobayashi K, Barrandon Y. Location of stem cells of human hair folli-cles by clonal analysis. Cell 1994;76:1063–73.

12. Guillem PG. How to make a Barrett esophagus: pathophysiology of columnar metaplasia of the esophagus. Dig Dis Sci 2005;50:415–24.

13. Ahnen DJ, Poulsom R, Stamp GW, et al. The ulceration-associated cell lineage (UACL) reiterates the Brunner's gland differentiation programme but acquires the proliferative organization of the gastric gland. J Pathol 1994;173:317–26.

14. Coad RA, Woodman AC, Warner PJ, et al. On the histogenesis of Barrett's oesoph-agus and its associated squamous islands: a three-dimensional study of their morphological relationship with native oesophageal gland ducts. J Pathol 2005; 206:388–94.

15. Chang CL, Lao-Sirieix P, Save V, et al. Retinoic acid-induced glandular differen-tiation of the oesophagus. Gut 2007;56:906–17.

16. Abdulnour-Nakhoul S, Nakhoul NL, Wheeler SA, et al. Characterization of esoph-ageal submucosal glands in pig tissue and cultures. Dig Dis Sci 2007;52: 3054–65.

17. Leedham SJ, Preston SL, McDonald SA, et al. Individual crypt genetic heteroge-neity and the origin of metaplastic glandular epithelium in human Barrett's oesophagus. Gut 2008;57(8):1041–8.

18. Paulson TG, Xu L, Sanchez C, et al. Neosquamous epithelium does not typically arise from Barrett's epithelium. Clin Cancer Res 2006;12:1701–6.

19. Sarosi G, Brown G, Jaiswal K, et al. Bone marrow progenitor cells contribute to esophageal regeneration and metaplasia in a rat model of Barrett's esophagus. Dis Esophagus 2008;21:43–50.

20. Houghton J, Stoicov C, Nomura S, et al. Gastric cancer originating from bone marrow-derived cells. Science 2004;306:1568–71.

21. Miyashita T, Ohta T, Fujimura T, et al. Duodenal juice stimulates oesophageal stem cells to induce Barrett's oesophagus and oesophageal adenocarcinoma in rats. Oncol Rep 2006;15:1469–75.

22. McDonald SA, Greaves LC, Gutierrez-Gonzalez L, et al. Mechanisms of field cancerization in the human stomach: the expansion and spread of mutated gastric stem cells. Gastroenterology 2008;134:500–10.

23. Bremner CG, Lynch VP, Ellis FH Jr. Barrett's esophagus: congenital or acquired? An experimental study of esophageal mucosal regeneration in the dog. Surgery 1970;68:209–16.
24. Kahrilas PJ, Dodds WJ, Hogan WJ, et al. Esophageal peristaltic dysfunction in peptic esophagitis. Gastroenterology 1986;91:897–904.
25. Tharalson EF, Martinez SD, Garewal HS, et al. Relationship between rate of change in acid exposure along the esophagus and length of Barrett's epithelium. Am J Gastroenterol 2002;97:851–6.
26. Peters FT, Ganesh S, Kuipers EJ, et al. Endoscopic regression of Barrett's oesophagus during omeprazole treatment; a randomised double blind study. Gut 1999;45:489–94.
27. Peters FT, Ganesh S, Kuipers EJ, et al. Effect of elimination of acid reflux on epithelial cell proliferative activity of Barrett esophagus. Scand J Gastroenterol 2000;35:1238–44.
28. Hillman LC, Chiragakis L, Shadbolt B, et al. Effect of proton pump inhibitors on markers of risk for high-grade dysplasia and oesophageal cancer in Barrett's oesophagus. Aliment Pharmacol Ther 2008;27:321–6.
29. Lao-Sirieix P, Roy A, Worrall C, et al. Effect of acid suppression on molecular predictors for esophageal cancer. Cancer Epidemiol Biomarkers Prev 2006; 15:288–93.
30. de Jonge PJ, Siersema PD, van Breda SG, et al. Proton pump inhibitor therapy in gastro-oesophageal reflux disease decreases the oesophageal immune response but does not reduce the formation of DNA adducts. Aliment Pharmacol Ther 2008;28(1):127–36.
31. Tobey NA, Reddy SP, Keku TO, et al. Mechanisms of HCl-induced lowering of intracellular pH in rabbit esophageal epithelial cells. Gastroenterology 1993; 105:1035–44.
32. Lao-Sirieix P, Corovic A, Jankowski J, et al. Physiological and molecular analysis of acid loading mechanisms in squamous and columnar-lined esophagus. Dis Esophagus 2007; doi:10.1111/j.1442-2050.2007.00796.x.
33. Tobey NA, Cragoe EJ Jr, Orlando RC. HCl-induced cell edema in rabbit esophageal epithelium: a bumetanide-sensitive process. Gastroenterology 1995;109: 414–21.
34. Orlando RC, Bryson JC, Powell DW. Mechanisms of H+ injury in rabbit esophageal epithelium. Am J Physiol 1984;246:G718–24.
35. Namiot Z, Sarosiek J, Marcinkiewicz M, et al. Declined human esophageal mucin secretion in patients with severe reflux esophagitis. Dig Dis Sci 1994; 39:2523–9.
36. Guillem P, Billeret V, Buisine MP, et al. Mucin gene expression and cell differentiation in human normal, premalignant and malignant esophagus. Int J Cancer 2000;88:856–61.
37. Tobey NA, Reddy SP, Khalbuss WE, et al. Na(+)-dependent and -independent Cl-/HCO3- exchangers in cultured rabbit esophageal epithelial cells. Gastroenterology 1993;104:185–95.
38. Hollwarth ME, Smith M, Kvietys PR, et al. Esophageal blood flow in the cat: normal distribution and effects of acid perfusion. Gastroenterology 1986;90:622–7.
39. Meyer W, Vollmar F, Bar W. Barrett-esophagus following total gastrectomy: a contribution to its pathogenesis. Endoscopy 1979;11:121–6.
40. Gutschow CA, Vallbohmer D, Stolte M, et al. Adenocarcinoma developing in de novo Barrett's mucosa in the remnant esophagus after esophagectomy: clinical and molecular assessment. Dis Esophagus 2008;21:E6–8.

41. Seto Y, Kobori O. Role of reflux oesophagitis and acid in the development of columnar epithelium in the rat oesophagus. Br J Surg 1993;80:467–70.
42. Kivilaakso E, Fromm D, Silen W. Effect of bile salts and related compounds on isolated esophageal mucosa. Surgery 1980;87:280–5.
43. Eda A, Osawa H, Satoh K, et al. Aberrant expression of CDX2 in Barrett's epithelium and inflammatory esophageal mucosa. J Gastroenterol 2003;38:14–22.
44. Pera M, Pera M, de Bolos C, et al. Duodenal-content reflux into the esophagus leads to expression of Cdx2 and Muc2 in areas of squamous epithelium in rats. J Gastrointest Surg 2007;11:869–74.
45. Hu Y, Williams VA, Gellersen O, et al. The pathogenesis of Barrett's esophagus: secondary bile acids upregulate intestinal differentiation factor CDX2 expression in esophageal cells. J Gastrointest Surg 2007;11:827–34.
46. Kazumori H, Ishihara S, Rumi MA, et al. Bile acids directly augment caudal related homeobox gene Cdx2 expression in oesophageal keratinocytes in Barrett's epithelium. Gut 2006;55:16–25.
47. Lechner S, Muller-Ladner U, Schlottmann K, et al. Bile acids mimic oxidative stress induced upregulation of thioredoxin reductase in colon cancer cell lines. Carcinogenesis 2002;23:1281–8.
48. Wilson KT, Fu S, Ramanujam KS, et al. Increased expression of inducible nitric oxide synthase and cyclooxygenase-2 in Barrett's esophagus and associated adenocarcinomas. Cancer Res 1998;58:2929–34.
49. Winter JW, Paterson S, Scobie G, et al. N-nitrosamine generation from ingested nitrate via nitric oxide in subjects with and without gastroesophageal reflux. Gastroenterology 2007;133:164–74.
50. Clemons NJ, McColl KE, Fitzgerald RC. Nitric oxide and acid induce double-strand DNA breaks in Barrett's esophagus carcinogenesis via distinct mechanisms. Gastroenterology 2007;133:1198–209.
51. Jang TJ, Min SK, Bae JD, et al. Expression of cyclooxygenase 2, microsomal prostaglandin E synthase 1, and EP receptors is increased in rat oesophageal squamous cell dysplasia and Barrett's metaplasia induced by duodenal contents reflux. Gut 2004;53:27–33.
52. Jolly AJ, Wild CP, Hardie LJ. Acid and bile salts induce DNA damage in human oesophageal cell lines. Mutagenesis 2004;19:319–24.
53. Feagins LA, Zhang HY, Zhang X, et al. Mechanisms of oxidant production in esophageal squamous cell and Barrett's cell lines. Am J Physiol Gastrointest Liver Physiol 2008;294(2):G411–7.
54. Dvorak K, Chavarria M, Payne CM, et al. Activation of the interleukin-6/STAT3 antiapoptotic pathway in esophageal cells by bile acids and low pH: relevance to barrett's esophagus. Clin Cancer Res 2007;13:5305–13.
55. Tselepis C, Perry I, Dawson C, et al. Tumour necrosis factor-alpha in Barrett's oesophagus: a potential novel mechanism of action. Oncogene 2002;21:6071–81.
56. Moons LM, Kusters JG, Bultman E, et al. Barrett's oesophagus is characterized by a predominantly humoral inflammatory response. J Pathol 2005;207:269–76.
57. Fitzgerald RC, Onwuegbusi BA, Bajaj-Elliott M, et al. Diversity in the oesophageal phenotypic response to gastro-oesophageal reflux: immunological determinants. Gut 2002;50:451–9.
58. Fitzgerald RC, Abdalla S, Onwuegbusi BA, et al. Inflammatory gradient in Barrett's oesophagus: implications for disease complications. Gut 2002;51:316–22.
59. Johansson M, Denardo DG, Coussens LM. Polarized immune responses differentially regulate cancer development. Immunol Rev 2008;222:145–54.

60. Moons LM, Kusters JG, van Delft JH, et al. A pro-inflammatory genotype predisposes to Barrett's esophagus. Carcinogenesis 2008;29(5):926–31.
61. Rabinovitch PS, Longton G, Blount PL, et al. Predictors of progression in Barrett's esophagus III: baseline flow cytometric variables. Am J Gastroenterol 2001;96:3071–83.
62. Chaves P, Crespo M, Ribeiro C, et al. Chromosomal analysis of Barrett's cells: demonstration of instability and detection of the metaplastic lineage involved. Mod Pathol 2007;20:788–96.
63. Meltzer SJ, Yin J, Manin B, et al. Microsatellite instability occurs frequently and in both diploid and aneuploid cell populations of Barrett's-associated esophageal adenocarcinomas. Cancer Res 1994;54:3379–82.
64. Reid BJ, Haggitt RC, Rubin CE, et al. Barrett's esophagus: correlation between flow cytometry and histology in detection of patients at risk for adenocarcinoma. Gastroenterology 1987;93:1–11.
65. Fennerty MB, Sampliner RE, Way D, et al. Discordance between flow cytometric abnormalities and dysplasia in Barrett's esophagus. Gastroenterology 1989;97: 815–20.
66. Galipeau PC, Li X, Blount PL, et al. NSAIDs modulate CDKN2A, TP53, and DNA content risk for progression to esophageal adenocarcinoma. PLoS Med 2007;4: 342–54.
67. Gleeson CM, Sloan JM, McGuigan JA, et al. Ubiquitous somatic alterations at microsatellite alleles occur infrequently in Barrett's-associated esophageal adenocarcinoma. Cancer Res 1996;56:259–63.
68. Olliver JR, Hardie LJ, Dexter S, et al. DNA damage levels are raised in Barrett's oesophageal mucosa relative to the squamous epithelium of the oesophagus. Biomarkers 2003;8:509–21.
69. Olliver JR, Hardie LJ, Gong Y, et al. Risk factors, DNA damage, and disease progression in Barrett's esophagus. Cancer Epidemiol Biomarkers Prev 2005; 14:620–5.
70. Fitzgerald RC. Molecular basis of Barrett's oesophagus and oesophageal adenocarcinoma. Gut 2006;55:1810–20.
71. Daniely Y, Liao G, Dixon D, et al. Critical role of p63 in the development of a normal esophageal and tracheobronchial epithelium. Am J Physiol Cell Physiol 2004;287:C171–81.
72. Geddert H, Kiel S, Heep HJ, et al. The role of p63 and deltaNp63 (p40) protein expression and gene amplification in esophageal carcinogenesis. Hum Pathol 2003;34:850–6.
73. Roman S, Petre A, Thepot A, et al. Downregulation of p63 upon exposure to bile salts and acid in normal and cancer esophageal cells in culture. Am J Physiol Gastrointest Liver Physiol 2007;293:G45–53.
74. Yamamoto H, Bai YQ, Yuasa Y. Homeodomain protein CDX2 regulates goblet-specific MUC2 gene expression. Biochem Biophys Res Commun 2003;300: 813–8.
75. Vallbohmer D, DeMeester SR, Peters JH, et al. Cdx-2 expression in squamous and metaplastic columnar epithelia of the esophagus. Dis Esophagus 2006; 19:260–6.
76. Moons LM, Bax DA, Kuipers EJ, et al. The homeodomain protein CDX2 is an early marker of Barrett's oesophagus. J Clin Pathol 2004;57:1063–8.
77. Silberg DG, Sullivan J, Kang E, et al. Cdx2 ectopic expression induces gastric intestinal metaplasia in transgenic mice. Gastroenterology 2002;122: 689–96.

78. Reid BJ, Sanchez CA, Blount PL, et al. Barrett's esophagus: cell cycle abnormalities in advancing stages of neoplastic progression. Gastroenterology 1993;105: 119–29.

79. Lao-Sirieix P, Brais R, Lovat L, et al. Cell cycle phase abnormalities do not account for disordered proliferation in Barrett's carcinogenesis. Neoplasia 2004;6:751–60.

80. Arber N, Lightdale C, Rotterdam H, et al. Increased expression of the cyclin D1 gene in Barrett's esophagus. Cancer Epidemiol Biomarkers Prev 1996;5:457–9.

81. Lu F, Gladden AB, Diehl JA. An alternatively spliced cyclin D1 isoform, cyclin D1b, is a nuclear oncogene. Cancer Res 2003;63:7056–61.

82. Umansky M, Yasui W, Hallak A, et al. Proton pump inhibitors reduce cell cycle abnormalities in Barrett's esophagus. Oncogene 2001;20:7987–91.

83. Lao-Sirieix P, Lovat L, Fitzgerald RC. Cyclin A immunocytology as a risk stratification tool for Barrett's esophagus surveillance. Clin Cancer Res 2007;13: 659–65.

84. Tannapfel A. Molecular findings in Barrett's epithelium. Dig Dis 2004;22:126–33.

85. Barrett MT, Sanchez CA, Prevo LJ, et al. Evolution of neoplastic cell lineages in Barrett oesophagus. Nat Genet 1999;22:106–9.

86. Segal F, Kaspary AP, Prolla JC, et al. p53 protein overexpression and p53 mutation analysis in patients with intestinal metaplasia of the cardia and Barrett's esophagus. Cancer Lett 2004;210:213–8.

87. Merola E, Mattioli E, Minimo C, et al. Immunohistochemical evaluation of pRb2/ p130, VEGF, EZH2, p53, p16, p21waf-1, p27, and PCNA in Barrett's esophagus. J Cell Physiol 2006;207:512–9.

88. Graeber TG, Osmanian C, Jacks T, et al. Hypoxia-mediated selection of cells with diminished apoptotic potential in solid tumours. Nature 1996;379:88–91.

89. Huang Y, Peters CJ, Fitzgerald RC, et al. Progressive silencing of p14ARF in oesophageal adenocarcinoma. J Cell Mol Med 2009;13(2):398–409.

90. Barrett MT, Sanchez CA, Galipeau PC, et al. Allelic loss of 9p21 and mutation of the CDKN2/p16 gene develop as early lesions during neoplastic progression in Barrett's esophagus. Oncogene 1996;13:1867–73.

91. Wong DJ, Paulson TG, Prevo LJ, et al. p16(INK4a) lesions are common, early abnormalities that undergo clonal expansion in Barrett's metaplastic epithelium. Cancer Res 2001;61:8284–9.

92. Maley CC, Galipeau PC, Li X, et al. Selectively advantageous mutations and hitchhikers in neoplasms: p16 lesions are selected in Barrett's esophagus. Cancer Res 2004;64:3414–27.

93. Maley CC, Galipeau PC, Finley JC, et al. Genetic clonal diversity predicts progression to esophageal adenocarcinoma. Nat Genet 2006;38:468–73.

94. Morales CP, Lee EL, Shay JW. In situ hybridization for the detection of telomerase RNA in the progression from Barrett's esophagus to esophageal adenocarcinoma. Cancer 1998;83:652–9.

95. Lord RV, Salonga D, Danenberg KD, et al. Telomerase reverse transcriptase expression is increased early in the Barrett's metaplasia, dysplasia, adenocarcinoma sequence. J Gastrointest Surg 2000;4:135–42.

96. Klump B, Hsieh CJ, Holzmann K, et al. Hypermethylation of the CDKN2/p16 promoter during neoplastic progression in Barrett's esophagus. Gastroenterology 1998;115:1381–6.

97. Hardie LJ, Darnton SJ, Wallis YL, et al. p16 expression in Barrett's esophagus and esophageal adenocarcinoma: association with genetic and epigenetic alterations. Cancer Lett 2005;217:221–30.

98. Vieth M, Schneider-Stock R, Rohrich K, et al. INK4a-ARF alterations in Barrett's epithelium, intraepithelial neoplasia and Barrett's adenocarcinoma. Virchows Arch 2004;445:135–41.

99. Clement G, Guilleret I, He B, et al. Epigenetic alteration of the Wnt inhibitory factor-1 promoter occurs early in the carcinogenesis of Barrett's esophagus. Cancer Sci 2008;99:46–53.

100. Kawakami K, Brabender J, Lord RV, et al. Hypermethylated APC DNA in plasma and prognosis of patients with esophageal adenocarcinoma. J Natl Cancer Inst 2000;92:1805–11.

101. Clement G, Braunschweig R, Pasquier N, et al. Alterations of the Wnt signaling pathway during the neoplastic progression of Barrett's esophagus. Oncogene 2006;25:3084–92.

102. Schlesinger Y, Straussman R, Keshet I, et al. Polycomb-mediated methylation on Lys27 of histone H3 pre-marks genes for de novo methylation in cancer. Nat Genet 2007;39:232–6.

103. Liu T, Zhang X, So CK, et al. Regulation of Cdx2 expression by promoter methylation, and effects of Cdx2 transfection on morphology and gene expression of human esophageal epithelial cells. Carcinogenesis 2007;28:488–96.

104. Jin Z, Mori Y, Yang J, et al. Hypermethylation of the nel-like 1 gene is a common and early event and is associated with poor prognosis in early-stage esophageal adenocarcinoma. Oncogene 2007;26:6332–40.

105. Jin Z, Hamilton JP, Yang J, et al. Hypermethylation of the AKAP12 promoter is a biomarker of Barrett's-associated esophageal neoplastic progression. Cancer Epidemiol Biomarkers Prev 2008;17:111–7.

Histology of Metaplasia and Dysplasia in Barrett's Esophagus

Lisa Yerian, MD[a,b,*]

KEYWORDS

• Barrett's • Dysplasia • Histology • Metaplasia • Diagnosis

In accordance with the American College of Gastroenterology definition of Barrett's esophagus, the diagnosis requires the identification of intestinal metaplasia on histologic examination.[1] Histologic evaluation of Barrett's esophagus has thus become an essential tool in the diagnosis of Barrett's esophagus and assessment of dysplasia.

NORMAL ESOPHAGEAL HISTOLOGY

The esophagus is comprised of four layers: the outermost serosa or adventitia, muscularis propria, submucosa, and a mucosal lining. The mucosa includes a nonkeratinizing stratified squamous epithelium, a supporting lamina propria, and the muscularis mucosae (**Fig. 1**). Indigenous mucus-secreting glands (cardiac glands) found within the lamina propria, particularly along the distal esophagus, produce neutral mucins and resemble the mucous glands of the stomach. The distal junction between squamous and columnar mucosa is termed the squamocolumnar junction or Z-line. Many adult patients have cardiac-type mucosa in the distal esophagus (up to 2–3 cm proximal to the gastroesophageal junction), and biopsy specimens procured from the distalmost esophagus frequently show inflamed cardiac-type mucosa.[2–7] Hence, the squamocolumnar junction does not necessarily coincide with the anatomic gastroesophageal junction (where the tubular esophagus joins the stomach).

[a] Hepatobiliary and Gastrointestinal Pathology, Cleveland Clinic Lerner College of Medicine, Cleveland, OH, USA
[b] Department of Anatomic Pathology, Cleveland Clinic, 9500 Euclid Avenue/L25, Cleveland, OH 44195, USA
* Corresponding author. Department of Pathology and Laboratory Medicine, Cleveland Clinic Foundation, 9500 Euclid Avenue/L25, Cleveland, OH 44195.
E-mail address: yerianl@ccf.org

Surg Oncol Clin N Am 18 (2009) 411–422
doi:10.1016/j.soc.2009.03.011
1055-3207/09/$ – see front matter © 2009 Elsevier Inc. All rights reserved.

surgonc.theclinics.com

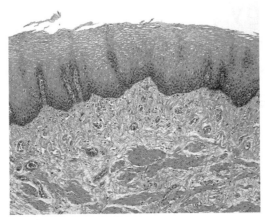

Fig. 1. Normal esophageal mucosa.

INTESTINAL METAPLASIA

Barrett's esophagus is the replacement of the normal stratified squamous epithelium of the esophagus with metaplastic columnar epithelium. Although precise endoscopic localization of the gastroesophageal junction may be difficult in some cases, if it is clear that a biopsy specimen has been procured from an endoscopically identified lesion in the tubular esophagus, then the identification of metaplastic intestinal epithelium is diagnostic of Barrett's esophagus.[1] Metaplastic intestinal-type columnar epithelium, variably termed "specialized," "intestinalized," or "intestinal-type" epithelium, is defined by the presence of acid mucin-containing goblet cells, and identification of goblet cells has thus become the accepted diagnostic histologic criterion of Barrett's esophagus. In the absence of intestinal metaplasia, a biopsy containing either cardiac- or fundic-type mucosa is not diagnostic of Barrett's esophagus. However, if the endoscopic findings are clearly those of Barrett's esophagus, then the absence of goblet cells may simply be a function of sampling error, particularly if few biopsies are taken.[8]

Goblet cells are epithelial cells with distended, mucin-filled cytoplasm and a barrel- or goblet-shaped configuration.[9] Goblet cells are interspersed among columnar cells and often exhibit a slightly more basophilic (ie, blue) cytoplasm than the adjacent columnar cells (**Fig. 2**). Goblet cells are positioned singly among a background of weakly eosinophilic columnar cells that may resemble either gastric foveolar cells or intestinal absorptive cells.[10] The distribution and relative proportion of goblet cells varies considerably among patients and specimens.[11] The gastric foveolar-type cells contain PAS-positive neutral mucins and are seen in combination with goblet cells in incomplete intestinal metaplasia, which is the more common form of intestinal metaplasia in Barrett's esophagus. Complete intestinal metaplasia is less common and contains variable numbers of goblet cells, intestinal absorptive-type cells, and sometimes even neuroendocrine cells and Paneth cells (complete intestinal metaplasia). An admixture of incomplete and complete intestinal metaplasia may also be seen.

Although in many cases intestinal metaplasia can be easily recognized on routine hematoxylin-eosin–stained slides, histochemical stains are a useful diagnostic adjunct in equivocal cases. These stains discriminate between goblet cells and the intervening columnar cells based on their mucin contents. Goblet cells contain both sialomucins and sulfated mucins that stain positively with alcian blue at pH 2.5, a characteristic that

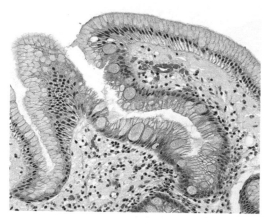

Fig. 2. Goblet cells.

allows histochemical distinction of goblet cells from adjacent columnar cells, which contain neutral mucins and are alcian blue negative (**Fig. 3**).[12] An alcian blue stain performed in conjunction with a periodic-acid–Schiff stain (PAS), can also be used to positively identify goblet cells, which stain blue due to their acidic mucins. The combined alcian blue/PAS stain highlights the contrast between the alcian-blue–positive goblet cells and strongly PAS-positive columnar cells (**Fig. 4**). These stains should always be interpreted with caution and in conjunction with morphologic interpretation, however, as gastric foveolar-type columnar cells may also contain alcian-blue–positive acid mucins, although the staining intensity is typically less than that seen in goblet cells. The identification of these alcian-blue–positive columnar cells (so-called "columnar blues") in the absence of goblet cells is insufficient for a definitive diagnosis of Barrett's esophagus.[13,14] Another helpful feature is that goblet cells are singly dispersed among columnar cells; a continuous row of alcian-blue–positive columnar cells is not diagnostic of intestinal metaplasia (**Fig. 5**). A diagnosis of intestinal metaplasia or Barrett's esophagus should be made only if the positively staining cells exhibit the appropriate morphologic features; recognition of the cell shape and staining quality is key to accurate diagnosis.

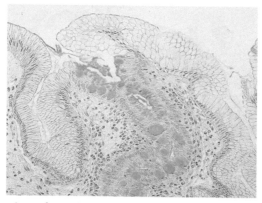

Fig. 3. Alcian blue stain performed at pH 2.5 highlights acid mucin-containing goblet cells but is negative in adjacent columnar cells.

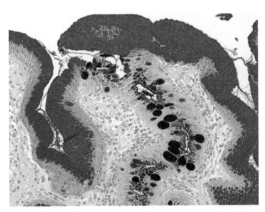

Fig. 4. Combined alcian blue/PAS staining technique provides sharp visual distinction between blue goblet cells and the adjacent pink columnar cells in Barrett's esophagus with incomplete metaplasia.

Barrett's esophagus is distinguished from several other types of glandular epithelium in the esophagus by the presence of intestinal metaplasia. For example, gastric-type mucosa may be sampled from a hiatal hernia, a focus of gastric heterotopia, or cardiac-like mucosa may all be sampled from the esophagus. Incidental foci of pancreatic acinar tissue, dubbed "pancreatic acinar metaplasia," are of no clinical significance.[15,16] Less common findings include esophageal superficial cardiac glands (often located in upper esophagus), ciliated columnar epithelium (embryologic remnant found in infants), or sebaceous glands. However, in the absence of intestinal metaplasia, any other types of glandular mucosa should not be interpreted as Barrett's esophagus.

INTESTINAL METAPLASIA OF THE GASTROESOPHAGEAL JUNCTION

Intestinal metaplasia is not unique to Barrett's esophagus. Intestinal metaplasia can also be seen in the stomach, including the gastric cardia, and is found near the

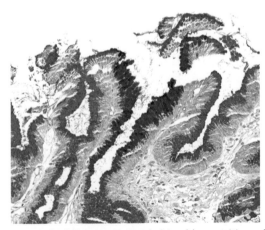

Fig. 5. Alcian blue/PAS stain highlights occasional alcian-blue–positive columnar cells, which should not be interpreted as representing intestinal metaplasia (compare with **Fig. 4**).

gastroesophageal junction in 9%–36% of patients who do not have an endoscopically identifiable segment of Barrett's mucosa.[17–19] However, the precise location of the gastroesophageal junction may be difficult to recognize during endoscopy, and it is not always possible to determine whether a biopsy derives from just above or just below the gastroesophageal junction. Furthermore, intestinal metaplasia of the upper stomach and distal esophagus may be histologically indistinguishable. According to the current American College of Gastroenterology definition of Barrett's esophagus, incidental goblet cells seen in biopsies from the junction in the absence of an endoscopic lesion do not fulfill the criteria for a diagnosis of Barrett's esophagus.[1]

DYSPLASIA IN BARRETT'S ESOPHAGUS

The importance of Barrett's esophagus lies in its premalignant nature, predisposing affected patients to the development of esophageal adenocarcinoma. Although all patients who have Barrett's esophagus are at increased risk for adenocarcinoma, some patients are at higher risk than others. Glandular epithelial dysplasia arising in Barrett's esophagus, particularly high-grade dysplasia, is a risk factor for development of synchronous or metachronous adenocarcinoma, based on mapping studies and prospective analyses.[20–26] Epithelial dysplasia may present as an endoscopically identifiable abnormality (eg, a nodule, erosion or polyp), but may also occur in the absence of an endoscopically identifiable lesion. Hence, thorough biopsy sampling is necessary to assess for dysplasia. In most institutions, patients who have Barrett's esophagus are placed in a surveillance program that involves four-quadrant biopsies taken every 2 cm throughout the length of the Barrett's segment with additional biopsies of any endoscopic lesions.[1,27]

Glandular epithelial dysplasia is defined as neoplastic epithelium confined within the basement membrane of the gland from which it arises.[28] In Barrett's esophagus, dysplasia is characterized by a combination of cytologic and architectural alterations and classified as either low grade or high grade based on the degree of the abnormality present. All biopsy specimens exhibiting Barrett's mucosa should be assessed for dysplasia, and possible histologic diagnostic categories include: negative for dysplasia, low-grade dysplasia, high-grade dysplasia, or epithelial alterations indefinite for dysplasia.

Negative for Dysplasia

A diagnosis of negative for dysplasia is applied when the epithelial cells are definitively not neoplastic (**Fig. 6**). In nondysplastic Barrett's mucosa, the glands present simple round or tubular shapes and are separated by intervening lamina propria. There is no architectural complexity (eg, irregularly shaped glands, glandular crowding, back-to-back or cribriform glands). The epithelial cells maintain their polarity, with nuclei oriented toward the basal membrane. Basal mitotic activity may be seen (as noted below), but mitotic figures are not seen at the mucosal surface, and abnormal mitotic figures are not seen. The epithelial cells exhibit maturation with decreased nuclear/cytoplasmic ratios as they progress from the base of the crypts toward the luminal surface.

When assessing for dysplasia in Barrett's esophagus, it is important for the pathologist to be aware that the glands at the base of Barrett's mucosa often show "baseline atypia." This term refers to nuclear enlargement, slight hyperchromasia and stratification, and increased mitotic activity seen at the base of the metaplastic crypts (**Fig. 7**). Thus, the absence of normal maturation as the cells progress toward the mucosal surface and the presence of cytologic atypia involving the surface epithelium are major

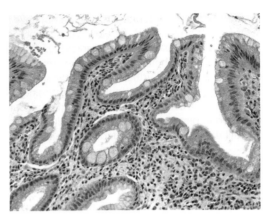

Fig. 6. Nondysplastic Barrett's mucosa.

diagnostic criteria for diagnosing dysplasia. That said, definitive identification of surface involvement is not always possible, and in certain cases a diagnosis of dysplasia is prudent in the absence of unequivocal surface involvement.[29] One should be very cautious when diagnosing dysplasia in this circumstance, though, and in most instances, when the only alterations are identified at the crypt bases and the cells mature normally towards the mucosal surface, a diagnosis of negative for dysplasia should be applied.

Low-Grade Dysplasia

Low-grade dysplasia shows either preservation or only minimal distortion of crypt architecture (**Fig. 8**). The involved glands remain separated by some fibrous stroma, with only mild gland crowding. There is no glandular complexity (eg, irregular, distorted, or cribriform glands). The cytology is characterized by closely packed cells with some (but not marked) nuclear enlargement, overlapping nuclei, variable hyperchromasia, and slightly irregular nuclear contours.[9,30,31] Overall, the epithelial cells retain their polarity, that is, the nuclei remain basally located with parallel nuclear axes oriented perpendicular to the basement membrane. Unlike nondysplastic Barrett's mucosa, dysplastic Barrett's mucosa demonstrates little or no maturation as the cells progress from the crypt bases to the luminal surface. The histologic features

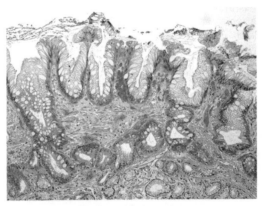

Fig. 7. Baseline atypia in glands at the base of Barrett's mucosa.

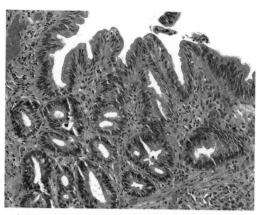

Fig. 8. In Barrett's esophagus with low-grade dysplasia, the neoplastic glands are only mildly crowded. The dysplastic epithelium exhibits enlarged, hyperchromatic and partially stratified nuclei with slightly irregular nuclear contours.

may recapitulate those seen in a typical tubular adenoma of the colon. Goblet cell numbers are often reduced, and dystrophic goblet cells may be present. One useful way to characterize low-grade dysplasia is epithelium that is unequivocally neoplastic but falls short of a diagnosis of high-grade dysplasia.

The natural history of low-grade dysplasia has not been well characterized, in part due to the high degree of interobserver variability related to the application of this diagnosis.[31,32] However, it is clear that there is an increased risk of progression to high-grade dysplasia or invasive adenocarcinoma in cases in which there is uniform agreement for a diagnosis of low-grade dysplasia.[33–35]

High-Grade Dysplasia

High-grade dysplasia exhibits more severe cytologic atypia and greater architectural complexity than does low-grade, but the cutoff between low-grade and high-grade dysplasia is difficult to define. There is no single picture of high-grade histology; rather, high-grade dysplasia occurs as a spectrum of histologic features that are unequivocally neoplastic with a greater degree of abnormality than low-grade dysplasia, but fall short of a diagnosis of carcinoma. Because of the varied histologic appearances, the diagnosis may be best learned not by seeing one picture of high-grade dysplasia, but rather by seeing a large number of cases demonstrating a wide spectrum of histologic lesions. High-grade dysplasia also exhibits more crypt architectural complexity with irregular, branched, and/or cribriform glands. The glands are usually more crowded than in nondysplastic mucosa or low-grade dysplasia, with only scant or absent intervening stroma separating glands (**Fig. 9**). The glands may exhibit a back-to-back pattern if they are very closely packed. High-grade dysplasia usually exhibits more nuclear crowding with nuclear stratification and prominent mitotic figures, which are often present at the mucosal surface (**Fig. 10**). The nuclear/cytoplasmic ratio is increased in the involved epithelium as compared with adjacent nondysplastic glands. Atypical mitotic figures may be seen. Normal maturation is not seen, and the surface epithelium is very similar to that seen deeper in the crypts in terms of nuclear-to-cytoplasmic ratio, nuclear size, and hyperchromasia.

Although high-grade dysplasia is the widely recognized precursor lesion for esophageal adenocarcinoma, it is not clear how often or how rapidly high-grade dysplasia

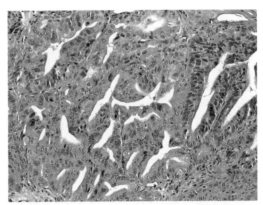

Fig. 9. In high grade dysplasia the neoplastic glands are irregularly shaped and are more crowded, separated only by thin strands of fibrovascular tissue.

progresses to cancer. In one prospective study of patients with a single focus of high-grade dysplasia with long-term follow-up (141), 53% of subjects developed either multifocal high-grade dysplasia or invasive carcinoma between 17 and 35 months of follow-up.[36] In contrast, in one large study of subjects with Barrett-related high-grade dysplasia without concurrent cancer, only 16% of subjects developed carcinoma during a mean surveillance period of 7.3 years.[37] In some cases, the distinction between high-grade dysplasia and intramucosal adenocarcinoma (defined by the penetration of neoplastic cells through the basement membrane to infiltrate into the lamina propria or muscularis mucosae) may be difficult, particularly in a biopsy specimen (**Fig. 11**).[38,39]

Indefinite for Dysplasia

As a rule, the diagnosis of "indefinite for dysplasia" is reserved for cases that are neither unequivocally dysplastic (neoplastic) nor definitively negative for dysplasia (nonneoplastic). Although this diagnostic category should not be overused, there are many situations in which the diagnosis of "indefinite for dysplasia" is not only appropriate but prudent. For example, many patients with Barrett's esophagus suffer

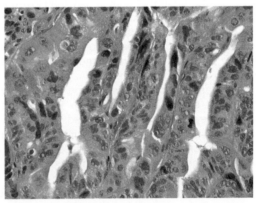

Fig. 10. The cytologic features of high-grade dysplasia include a greater degree of nuclear enlargement, pleomorphism, and hyperchromasia. There is often loss of polarity, and mitotic figures may be numerous, especially in reactive or regenerative epithelium.

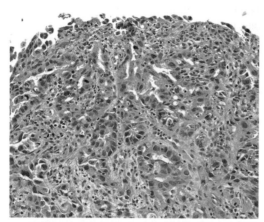

Fig. 11. This complex proliferation of neoplastic glands presents striking cytologic atypia and indicates at least high-grade dysplasia in Barrett's esophagus. The glandular profiles are jagged and irregular, and the basement membrane is difficult to identify in some areas.

from ongoing gastroesophageal reflux, and the associated inflammation and mucosal injury can result in epithelial cell changes that may be difficult to distinguish from dysplasia. Therefore one should always be cautious when making a diagnosis of dysplasia in the presence of active inflammation or mucosal erosion, and the indefinite category is often employed in this setting (**Fig. 12**). If the abnormalities could possibly represent florid regeneration, an express diagnosis of dysplasia is unsuitable. It is worth noting, however, that in cases in which the alterations are unequivocally non-neoplastic, a diagnosis of "indefinite" is neither necessary nor appropriate.

Although hyperchromasia and nuclear pleomorphism may be seen in dysplastic or reparative nuclei, the epithelial changes due to repair tend to be less severe and more uniform, with cells resembling their neighbors within the same crypt or in adjacent crypts. However, discrimination between reactive and neoplastic alterations is often not straightforward, and in such cases a diagnosis of "epithelial alterations indefinite for dysplasia" is appropriate. This diagnosis indicates that the histologic changes are neither unequivocally neoplastic ("positive for dysplasia") nor clearly reactive ("negative for dysplasia"). A period of antireflux therapy followed by

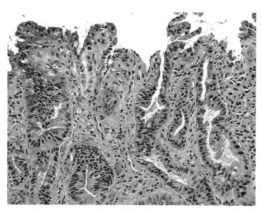

Fig. 12. In this case there is some hyperchromasia, but the surface epithelium is denuded and, where present, does not show clear neoplastic features.

re-biopsy is often helpful in confirming or excluding dysplasia in such cases. The diagnosis of indefinite may also be employed when the architectural or cytologic features are obscured by fixation, sectioning or staining artifacts, poor orientation, or when the findings fall quantitatively or qualitatively short of a definitive diagnosis of dysplasia.

COMPLICATING FACTORS

The histologic diagnosis of Barrett's dysplasia can be challenging due to sampling error, observer variation, and difficulty in histologic interpretation, and these problems complicate patient management. Although dysplasia can be diffusely present throughout a segment of Barrett's mucosa, in some cases the dysplastic changes are quite focal.[40] Small dysplastic foci may not be sampled despite using a rigorous endoscopic sampling technique. Similarly, a biopsy diagnosis of dysplasia does not exclude the presence of a more significant lesion. Indeed, up to 40% of patients with a biopsy diagnosis of high-grade dysplasia in the absence of a grossly recognizable lesion are found to have adenocarcinoma at esophagectomy.[41]

The significant interobserver variation in the diagnosis of Barrett's-related dysplasia has been illustrated.[31,32,42] Particularly problematic is the separation of negative, indefinite, and low-grade dysplasia, and the diagnosis of suboptimal biopsy material.[31,32,42] Because of the difficulty pathologists face in this arena, multiple opinions should be sought on difficult cases, and the diagnosis of dysplasia should be confirmed by a pathologist experienced in Barrett's esophagus before aggressive therapy is contemplated.

REFERENCES

1. Wang KK, Sampliner RE. Updated guidelines for the diagnosis, surveillance, and therapy of Barrett's esophagus. Practice Parameters Committee of the American College of Gastroenterology. Am J Gastroenterol 2008;103(3):788–97.
2. Chandrasoma P. Controversies of the cardiac mucosa and Barrett's oesophagus. Histopathology 2005;46:361–73.
3. Chandrasoma PT, Der R, Ma Y, et al. Histology of the gastroesophageal junction: an autopsy study. Am J Surg Pathol 2000;24:402–9.
4. Chandrasoma PT, Lokuhetty DM, Demeester TR, et al. Definition of histopathologic changes in gastroesophageal reflux disease. Am J Surg Pathol 2000;24:344–51.
5. Oberg S, Peters JH, DeMeester TR, et al. Inflammation and specialized intestinal metaplasia of cardiac mucosa is a manifestation of gastroesophageal reflux disease. Ann Surg 1997;226:522–30.
6. Odze RD. Pathology of the gastroesophageal junction. Semin Diagn Pathol 2005; 22(4):256–65.
7. Sarbia M, Donner A, Gabbert HE. Histopathology of the gastroesophageal junction: a study on 36 operation specimens. Am J Surg Pathol 2002;26:1207–12.
8. Harrison R, Perry I, Haddadin W, et al. Detection of intestinal metaplasia in Barrett's esophagus: an observational comparator study suggests the need for a minimum of eight biopsies. Am J Gastroenterol 2007;102:1154–61.
9. Goldblum JR. Barrett's esophagus and Barrett's-related dysplasia. Mod Pathol 2003;16:316–24.
10. Levine DS, Rubin CE, Reid BJ, et al. Specialized metaplastic columnar epithelium in Barrett's esophagus. A comparative transmission electron microscopic study. Lab Invest 1989;60:418–32.

11. Qualman SJ, Murray RD, McClung HJ, et al. Intestinal metaplasia is age related in Barrett's esophagus. Arch Pathol Lab Med 1990;114:1236–40.
12. Haggitt RC, Reid BJ, Rabinovitch PS, et al. Barrett's esophagus. Correlation between mucin histochemistry, flow cytometry, and histologic diagnosis for predicting increased cancer risk. Am J Pathol 1988;131:53–61.
13. Chen YY, Wang HH, Antonioli DA, et al. Significance of acid-mucin-positive non-goblet columnar cells in the distal esophagus and gastroesophageal junction. Hum Pathol 1999;30:1488–95.
14. Offner FA, Lewin KJ, Weinstein WM. Metaplastic columnar cells in Barrett's esophagus: a common and neglected cell type. Hum Pathol 1996;27:885–9.
15. Krishnamurthy S, Dayal Y. Pancreatic metaplasia in Barrett's esophagus. An immunohistochemical study. Am J Surg Pathol 1995;19:1172–80.
16. Wang HH, Zeroogian JM, Spechler SJ, et al. Prevalence and significance of pancreatic acinar metaplasia at the gastroesophageal junction. Am J Surg Pathol 1996;20:1507–10.
17. Johnston MH, Hammond AS, Laskin W, et al. The prevalence and clinical characteristics of short segments of specialized intestinal metaplasia in the distal esophagus on routine endoscopy. Am J Gastroenterol 1996;91:1507–11.
18. Nandurkar S, Talley NJ, Martin CJ, et al. Short segment Barrett's oesophagus: prevalence, diagnosis and associations. Gut 1997;40:710–5.
19. Trudgill NJ, Suvarna SK, Kapur KC, et al. Intestinal metaplasia at the squamocolumnar junction in patients attending for diagnostic gastroscopy. Gut 1997;41:585–9.
20. Haggitt RC. Barrett's esophagus, dysplasia, and adenocarcinoma. Hum Pathol 1994;25:982–93.
21. Hameeteman W, Tytgat GN, Houthoff HJ, et al. Barrett's esophagus: development of dysplasia and adenocarcinoma. Gastroenterology 1989;96:1249–56.
22. Hamilton SR, Smith RR. The relationship between columnar epithelial dysplasia and invasive adenocarcinoma arising in Barrett's esophagus. Am J Clin Pathol 1987;87:301–12.
23. Oberg S, Wenner J, Johansson J, et al. Barrett esophagus: risk factors for progression to dysplasia and adenocarcinoma. Ann Surg 2005;242:49–54.
24. Reid BJ, Weinstein WM, Lewin KJ, et al. Endoscopic biopsy can detect high-grade dysplasia or early adenocarcinoma in Barrett's esophagus without grossly recognizable neoplastic lesions. Gastroenterology 1988;94:81–90.
25. Schmidt HG, Riddell RH, Walther B, et al. Dysplasia in Barrett's esophagus. J Cancer Res Clin Oncol 1985;110:145–52.
26. Smith RR, Hamilton SR, Boitnott JK, et al. The spectrum of carcinoma arising in Barrett's esophagus. A clinicopathologic study of 26 patients. Am J Surg Pathol 1984;8:563–73.
27. Lunedei V, Bazzoli F, Pozzato P, et al. Endoscopic surveillance in Barrett's esophagus. Minerva Gastroenterol Dietol 2002;48:63–71.
28. Riddell RH, Goldman H, Ransohoff DF, et al. Dysplasia in inflammatory bowel disease: standardized classification with provisional clinical applications. Hum Pathol 1983;14:931–68.
29. Lomo LC, Blount PL, Sanchez CA, et al. Crypt dysplasia with surface maturation: a clinical, pathologic, and molecular study of a Barrett's esophagus cohort. Am J Surg Pathol 2006;30:423–35.
30. Goldblum JR, Lauwers GY. Dysplasia arising in Barrett's esophagus: diagnostic pitfalls and natural history. Semin Diagn Pathol 2002;19:12–9.
31. Montgomery E, Bronner MP, Goldblum JR, et al. Reproducibility of the diagnosis of dysplasia in Barrett esophagus: a reaffirmation. Hum Pathol 2001;32:368–78.

32. Reid BJ, Haggitt RC, Rubin CE, et al. Observer variation in the diagnosis of dysplasia in Barrett's esophagus. Hum Pathol 1988;19:166–78.
33. Dulai GS, Shekelle PG, Jensen DM, et al. Dysplasia and risk of further neoplastic progression in a regional Veterans Administration Barrett's cohort. Am J Gastroenterol 2005;100:775–83.
34. Lim CH, Treanor D, Dixon MF, et al. Low-grade dysplasia in Barrett's esophagus has a high risk of progression. Endoscopy 2007;39:581–7.
35. Skacel M, Petras RE, Gramlich TL, et al. The diagnosis of low-grade dysplasia in Barrett's esophagus and its implications for disease progression. Am J Gastroenterol 2000;95:3383–7.
36. Weston AP, Sharma P, Topalovski M, et al. Long-term follow-up of Barrett's high-grade dysplasia. Am J Gastroenterol 2000;95:1888–93.
37. Schnell TG, Sontag SJ, Chejfec G, et al. Long-term nonsurgical management of Barrett's esophagus with high-grade dysplasia. Gastroenterology 2001;120:1607–19.
38. Ormsby AH, Petras RE, Henricks WH, et al. Observer variation in the diagnosis of superficial oesophageal adenocarcinoma. Gut 2002;51:671–6.
39. Rice TW, Mendelin JE, Goldblum JR. Barrett's esophagus: pathologic considerations and implications for treatment. Semin Thorac Cardiovasc Surg 2005;17:292–300.
40. Dar MS, Goldblum JR, Rice TW, et al. Can extent of high grade dysplasia in Barrett's oesophagus predict the presence of adenocarcinoma at oesophagectomy? Gut 2003;52:486–9.
41. Falk GW, Rice TW, Goldblum JR, et al. Jumbo biopsy forceps protocol still misses unsuspected cancer in Barrett's esophagus with high-grade dysplasia. Gastrointest Endosc 1999;49:170–6.
42. Kerkhof M, van Dekken H, Steyerberg EW, et al. Grading of dysplasia in Barrett's oesophagus: substantial interobserver variation between general and gastrointestinal pathologists. Histopathology 2007;50:920–7.

Improving Screening Practices for Barrett's Esophagus

Nicholas J. Shaheen, MD, MPH[a,b,*], Lena B. Palmer, MD[c]

KEYWORDS

- Barrett's esophagus • Screening
- Gastroesophageal reflux disease (GERD)
- Esophageal adenocarcinoma • Epidemiology

An effective screening program has several seminal characteristics: (1) an identifiable population at risk, (2) a reliable, tolerable, and cost-effective screening examination, (3) effective treatment for early-stage disease, and (4) evidence of improved outcomes outweighing harms.[1,2] In order to improve screening practices for Barrett's esophagus (BE), one must examine the effectiveness of the current system in light of these four components. By reviewing the evidence behind screening practices for BE within each component, one quickly realizes how much data are lacking to substantiate endoscopic screening practices for BE.

IDENTIFIABLE POPULATION AT RISK FOR DISEASE

One key concern about endoscopic screening programs for BE is that defining a population at sufficiently high risk for the disease to be prevented (adenocarcinoma of the esophagus) is difficult. Current recommendations make little effort to stratify risk based on demographic or symptom-specific criteria, leaving the field to provide widespread screening to patients who have low risk for BE and even lower risk for adenocarcinoma of the esophagus (ACE). Emerging evidence has helped refine current risk factors and add new potential risk factors, but this information has yet to be

This work was supported by NIH grant R03DK75842.
[a] Departments of Medicine and Epidemiology, Schools of Medicine and Public Health, CB#7080, UNC-CH, Chapel Hill, NC 27599-7080, USA
[b] University of North Carolina Center for Esophageal Diseases and Swallowing, University of North Carolina School of Medicine, CB#7080, UNC-CH, Chapel Hill, NC 27599-7080, USA
[c] Division of Gastroenterology and Hepatology, University of North Carolina Center for Esophageal Diseases and Swallowing, University of North Carolina School of Medicine, 4162R Bioinformatics Bldg, 130 Mason Farm Road, Chapel Hill, NC 27599-7080, USA
* Corresponding author. UNC Center for Esophageal Diseases and Swallowing, University of North Carolina School of Medicine, CB#7080, UNC-CH, Chapel Hill, NC 27599-7080.
E-mail address: nshaheen@med.unc.edu (N. J. Shaheen).

incorporated into practice guidelines for screening, and may require years to shape clinical practice.

Current Suggested Screening Populations

Several major gastroenterology societies have endorsed screening patients with chronic gastroesophageal reflux disease (GERD), but further specification by patient characteristics varies by recommending society. The American College of Gastroenterology (ACG), American Society of Gastrointestinal Endoscopists (ASGE) and the American Gastroenterological Association (AGA) note associations between BE and the severity of GERD symptoms, the length of GERD diagnosis, and the race, gender, and age of the patient.[3-5] The AGA suggests that gastroenterologists consider screening white male patients over the age of fifty who have chronic, longstanding GERD,[5] and the ASGE adds that patients who have frequent heartburn (several times per week) and nocturnal symptoms should be considered as well.[4] The ACG recently changed its recommendations from screening patients with chronic GERD to screening at the discretion of the physician in high-risk patients.[6]

The problem with chronic reflux symptoms as an entry criterion for a screening program for ACE is that it is a neither sensitive nor specific marker for the disease. Cohort and case-control studies demonstrate that almost half of those who develop cancer report no antecedent chronic heartburn.[7,8] Among those who do have heartburn, the risk of developing ACE, although elevated compared with the general public, is still less than 1 in 1,000.[9]

All societies agree that only patients who would survive the treatment of any neoplasia isolated from a screening examination should be considered for screening. This caveat to screening was more significant when the only existing treatment for ACE was surgical resection via esophagectomy. Given the high morbidity and potential mortality from this procedure,[10] it was important to consider the patient's clinical status before proceeding with any screening examination. Emerging therapies, discussed below, have broadened the screening population by providing less morbid treatment options capable of benefiting a wider range of patients.

Risk factors for Barrett's esophagus

Though the current screening population consists mostly of patients who have chronic heartburn, there are several other demographic characteristics of subjects that increase the likelihood of BE, including increasing age, white race, and increasing duration and frequency of GERD symptoms. Recent data have also suggested that obesity, especially truncal obesity, and smoking may increase the risk of BE in GERD patients.[11,12] A large proportion of BE occurs in patients without reflux symptoms and a large proportion of ACE occurs in patients without BE.[13] These findings limit the utility of any screening program that solely targets patients with GERD.

Age

Unlike other screening programs, such as colorectal cancer and breast cancer, that set defined age limits for the initiation of screening, major recommending organizations have been reluctant to recommend a firm age at which to begin or end screening for BE or ACE. Some authorities have suggested initial endoscopy at age 50 in white men, and indeed almost all cost-effectiveness analyses of screening programs have used Markov models based on this age.[14-17] Studies of cancer risk in Barrett's esophagus demonstrate that cancer in the setting of BE is almost exclusively a disease of older adults, with an average age at time of diagnosis of 60+ years.[18-25]

Duration and severity of reflux symptoms

The term "chronic GERD" in the definition of the current screening population refers to the length of time the patient has suffered from reflux symptoms. The ASGE proposed that patients who have symptoms of heartburn for greater than 5 years should be considered for screening, based on evidence that the rate of BE increases as the duration of symptoms increases.[26–28] In one study of reflux disease and the presence of BE in a community cohort, the odds of having BE was three times greater in subjects who had heartburn symptoms for 1–5 years versus those who had symptoms for less than 1 year. In subjects who had symptoms for 10 years or more, the odds ratio was as high as 6.4.[29] Other cohort studies have also shown a correlation between BE and the frequency of reflux symptoms.[30] In one study of GERD symptoms and ACE,[7] a long duration of reflux symptoms combined with a high severity of disease increased the odds of ACE to 43.5 (95% CI, 18.3–103.5). This study only considered the association between reflux and ACE and did not control for the presence of BE.

Some researchers have demonstrated an inverse association between severity of reflux symptoms and BE, suggesting that the intestinal metaplasia may be a protective mechanism to decrease the sensation of acid exposure in the esophagus. Brandt and colleagues[31] showed that GERD subjects who were diagnosed with BE reported less severe reflux symptoms compared with GERD subjects who did not have BE, despite having higher and more prolonged exposure to an acid environment. This finding is consistent with other studies showing decreased acid sensitivity and decreased self-reported severity of reflux symptoms among subjects who have BE.[32,33]

Race and gender

Evidence from surgical resections of ACE arising in BE has shown that the risk of ACE overwhelmingly predominates in white men.[34–36] One study that examined risk of BE in Asian subjects who had GERD did show an elevated prevalence of BE in these other racial groups (5.2% for short- and long-segment BE),[37] suggesting that the association between ACE and white race seen in United States studies may be at least in part due to the demographics of the source population. Therefore, it is possible that screening recommendations should vary according to the distribution of race in the underlying population.

Medical and surgical therapy

The recommendations for screening patients who have GERD for the presence of BE have also included patients who have undergone surgical and medical antireflux treatments. Recently published data have shown a decreased risk of progression to high-grade dysplasia and ACE in subjects with successful antireflux surgery.[38] This is inconsistent with a meta-analysis showing no effect of surgical antireflux procedures upon the incidence of ACE in subjects who have BE.[39] Although some studies have shown that the use of H2 receptor antagonists and proton pump inhibitors decreases the length of a Barrett's esophagus segment,[40] the preponderance of data do not support this contention.[6] Weak evidence from retrospective studies suggests that PPI therapy may diminish the risk of progression to dysplasia.[41] However, until further data are available supporting a decreased ACE incidence via antireflux procedures or medical therapy, these patients should still be considered at increased risk of ACE.

Obesity and smoking

In addition to the risk factors mentioned above, obesity and smoking have emerged as risk factors for BE and ACE.[30,42–45] For obesity, this stems from a physiologic rationale that increased intraabdominal pressure due to obesity might increase the rate of hiatal hernias and the esophageal exposure to acid, thus increasing the potential for intestinal metaplasia. Studies have also examined the role that the obesity hormone leptin may play in the metaplasia–dysplasia–carcinoma pathway.[42] Other proinflammatory and proproliferative cytokines, such as IGF-I, are also elevated in obese subjects, suggesting that hormonal and mechanical factors might increase the risk of cancer in obese subjects.[46] Indeed, the continuous rise in incidence of ACE parallels an unprecedented epidemic of obesity. One group of researchers studied the interactions between obesity, smoking, and reflux symptoms and found that although reflux was still the predominant risk factor associated with BE, both obesity and smoking increased the risk of BE in addition to reflux alone.[30] In a surgical pathology series of resected ACE, smoking was found to quite prevalent among subjects who had adenocarcinoma (63% prevalence).[35] Conversely, one study of institutionalized intellectually challenged subjects who had high rates of reflux but low rates of smoking and alcohol use showed no difference in ACE rate versus a noninstitutionalized population, suggesting no evidence for increased risk from smoking.[25] Confusing the association is the finding that there is no difference between mean BMI among subjects who have GERD and subjects who have BE.[47] Clearly, obesity and smoking play a role in the development of BE and ACE, but the nature of this role, the interplay between the risk factors, and their individual impact on risk needs further definition.

Challenges to the Current Screening Population

Risk of Barrett's esophagus in patients without gastroesophageal reflux disease

One crucial patient population missing from the current target population is those who harbor BE without reflux symptoms. Two studies examining the rate of BE in subjects undergoing colonoscopy for reasons unrelated to esophageal symptoms showed a prevalence of BE in subjects who did not have reflux to be as high as those who had reflux symptoms.[48,49] Others have estimated that as much as half of the prevalent cases of BE exist in subjects who have no symptoms of reflux.[50] In a report of the prevalence of BE in a Swedish cohort, Ronkainen and colleagues[13] demonstrated an overall prevalence of BE of 1.6% in the general adult population, with 2.3% of BE occurring in subjects who had reflux symptoms, and 1.2% in subjects who did not have reflux. Until risk factors emerge that make it possible to identify BE patients who do not suffer from GERD, this population represents a large component of at-risk subjects who will continue to be missed by the current screening strategy.

Low risk of adenocarcinoma with nondysplastic Barrett's esophagus

There is a definite increase in risk of ACE in patients who have BE, but studies of mortality in subjects who had BE show that they rarely die from the cancer itself.[21,51,52] Cohort studies examining the risk of ACE in subjects who had BE have reported risk ratios as high as 30 to 125 times the general population[50,53] and an incidence of approximately 0.5% per year or 1 in 212 patient-years.[54] However, subjects who had BE have excess all-cause mortality compared with the general population [hazard ratio for death of 1.37 (95% CI, 1.12–1.66)], and less than 45% of this excess risk is due to death from ACE.[53] Two additional cohort studies have echoed the finding that ACE is a rare cause of death for subjects who had BE.[21,52] Because the goal of any screening program is to decrease disease-related mortality, it may be difficult to justify screening when the absolute risk for mortality from the disease may be only minimally elevated in the target population.

Risk of adenocarcinoma without Barrett's esophagus

Complicating our understanding of the disease progression from BE to ACE is the finding that a large proportion of subjects who develop ACE do not have a diagnosis of BE before the development of cancer. In one systematic review, only 5% of subjects undergoing resection of esophageal cancers had a prior diagnosis of BE.[55] Results from a Danish population-based cohort study spanning 20 years of observation revealed that only 32 cases of ACE were seen out of 60,000+ subjects, and only 34% of those cases occurred in subjects who had a diagnosis of BE greater than 1 year before the diagnosis of cancer.[56] This lack of recognition of a preexisting BE may be due to either underutilization of the screening test in GERD populations (one cannot receive a diagnosis of BE unless one undergoes endoscopy), or the insufficient presence of symptoms of GERD to warrant investigation, or the possibility that some cases of ACE occur without preceding BE. It is not entirely clear whether BE is always necessary as a precursor to ACE. However, a study of 79 subjects who had ACE who underwent chemotherapy showed a prechemotherapy prevalence of BE of 75%, and a postchemotherapy prevalence of 97%.[57] The high postchemotherapy prevalence of BE in this study suggests that the lack of BE seen in some patients who have ACE is due to carcinoma overgrowth of the underlying, preexisting BE mucosa. Further studies will be needed to confirm this hypothesis.

The problem of low absolute magnitude of risk

In all discussions of risk, the use of ratio measures of disease association such as risk ratios and odds ratios tend to distort the fact that the *absolute* risk for the development of adenocarcinoma of the esophagus (ACE) in the setting of chronic GERD symptoms is low. A Venn diagram of the relationships between GERD, BE, and ACE easily demonstrates the low yield from a screening program targeting ACE via GERD and BE (**Fig. 1**). Screening endoscopy performed in 10,000 adult patients over the age of 50 with chronic GERD has the potential to isolate between 500 and 1500 cases of BE[9] (410–1230 when the reported sensitivity of screening endoscopy is applied[58]). From the initial 10,000 endoscopies (and 80,000–160,000 biopsies taken during examination[59]), 6.5 prevalent cases of ACE might be expected, and an additional 2.5–7.5 cases per year would be added from surveillance of the 500–1500 patients found to have BE.[9] Put another way, less than 0.15% of the initial screened population is likely to have cancer or develop it within 1 year of the initial screen. These numbers are even lower when the only criterion for entry into a screening and surveillance program is longstanding GERD without other risk factors such as age, race, or gender.[3] These numbers also do not reflect the missed cases of BE in patients who do not have GERD, and future ACE that is destined to develop in patients without antecedent BE or GERD (areas denoted by question marks in **Fig. 1**). Finally, a portion of the prevalent cancers will likely be too advanced to be amenable to intervention, further decreasing the yield of the program for preventing death from cancer.

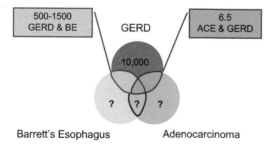

Fig. 1. Potential diagnostic yield of ACE when screening subjects over the age of 50 who have chronic GERD.

RELIABLE, TOLERABLE, COST-EFFECTIVE SCREENING EXAM

The second component of an effective screening program focuses on the screening test itself and whether it is reliable at identifying the preclinical lesion, tolerable and safe for patients, and cost-effective when implemented in a large population of patients. Unfortunately, endoscopic and histologic screening examinations for BE are fraught with variation in technique and interobserver reliability.

Endoscopy as a Screening Tool

Traditional white-light endoscopy is the most commonly used tool to assess for the presence of BE, but it imperfect when used in this setting. The visual identification of BE requires an accurate identification of both the lower esophageal sphincter and the gastroesophageal junction. This is particularly challenging in patients who have BE whereby there is reduced pressure in the lower esophageal sphincter,[60,61] and the common presence of a hiatal hernia. Further complicating the picture in some cases is the difficulty identifying Barrett's changes in concomitant erosive esophagitis. Overall, traditional endoscopy has been shown to have a sensitivity and positive predictive value (PPV) to detect BE of 82% and 34%, respectively, when used to screen white patients who have dyspepsia and/or suspected BE.[58] When the operating characteristics are examined in a population of African Americans who are less likely to have BE, the PPV falls to a dismal 15%.[58] A classification system called the Prague C&M criteria seeks to standardize the reporting of the endoscopic evaluation of the presence and extent of BE, and has shown good reliability among endoscopists with an overall reliability coefficient of 0.72 for the endoscopic recognition of BE segments 1 cm or greater.[62]

Biopsies are required to evaluate any abnormal-appearing mucosa, and various sizes of forceps, biopsy numbers, and length of affected mucosa will likely alter the yield from pathology, as well as the cost of examination. These operating characteristics cause the sensitivity of endoscopy to vary widely among practitioners, and by definition, to perform more poorly in patients who have short-segment BE where published reports of sensitivity of random biopsies to detect intestinal metaplasia is between 30%–50%.[63] The diagnostic yield of jumbo forceps versus standard forceps in the setting of screening is poorly understood.[6]

As for biopsy number and spacing, four-quadrant random biopsies are recommended every 1–2 cm of Barrett's–appearing mucosa, in addition to biopsies of all suspicious lesions. One study from Seattle found that biopsies every 2 cm missed 50% of identified cancers versus biopsies every 1 cm.[64] This observation helps inform the ACG recommendation for biopsies every 1 cm in patients who have high-grade dysplasia.[6] It is unclear whether the additional diagnostic yield of such an intensive protocol in screening subjects who have GERD (as opposed to surveillance of dysplasia) is high enough to justify the increased time and cost. Harrison and colleagues[59] attempted to identify the minimum number of biopsies needed to adequately identify intestinal metaplasia within biopsy specimens. The yield of intestinal metaplasia from endoscopy of subjects who had an average BE segment of 4 cm was 68% after eight biopsies; however, 16 biopsies were needed to achieve 100% yield. Additionally, the overall yield and effectiveness of screening endoscopy is lowered when one considers the reality that adherence to biopsy recommendations occurs in only about one half of all cases.[65,66]

Histologic Interpretation of Biopsy Specimens

Just as endoscopists cannot always agree upon the gross appearance of BE, the interobserver reliability from biopsy specimens shows a similar variation in agreement among pathologists for the diagnosis of dysplasia, because interobserver reliability depends upon the experience of the pathologist and the classification scheme that is used.[8] Although the presence of goblet cells can be reliably ascertained using standard staining techniques with periodic acid–Schiff alcian blue,[67] the interobserver variability in the diagnosis of dysplasia is high, and only marginally improves with education.[8,68]

Though biopsies are taken of any abnormal-appearing mucosa, there is some concern that BE will be missed when no biopsies are taken of normal-appearing mucosa. Lenglinger and colleagues[69] showed that there was no correlation between the endoscopic appearance of the mucosa and the presence of intestinal metaplasia in their series of 114 subjects undergoing endoscopy for GERD, suggesting that metaplastic cells could be present in macroscopically normal mucosa. The risk of malignant degeneration of intestinal metaplasia found in a normal-appearing GE junction is unknown, but is thought to be low.

Emerging Techniques

Several promising techniques, discussed in the article by Bergman and Sharma elsewhere in this issue, have been developed to increase the accuracy of endoscopic identification of BE, including magnification and chromoendoscopy,[63,70,71] narrow-band imaging,[72] capsule endoscopy,[73] and unsedated transnasal endoscopy.[74] Histologic confirmation will also improve as novel molecular markers for BE are incorporated into the pathologic evaluation of biopsy specimens. At this point, however, these advanced techniques are not widely available for use in the setting of screening, and endoscopists are not routinely trained to perform them. Their characteristics in a screening population have also not been established, nor has there been an analysis of benefit gained versus the incremental increase in cost and time of examination added by these new techniques.

EFFECTIVE TREATMENT OF EARLY-STAGE DISEASE

One of the greatest improvements to the treatment of adenocarcinoma of the esophagus (ACE) is the development of treatment modalities for early-stage disease that are highly effective, tolerable for patients, carry decreased morbidity and mortality compared with surgical resection, and may be able to decrease the risk of future ACE.

The traditional therapy for early stage cancer and high-grade dysplasia (HGD) was esophagectomy. Unfortunately, this surgery is associated with morbidity, and a substantial mortality when not done in select high volume centers.[10] Because a substantial proportion of those developing cancer have serious comorbidities, investigators have sought to develop methods of treating the neoplastic tissue without esophagectomy. Multiple modalities have been demonstrated effective in cohort studies, case series, or randomized trials of subjects who had HGD or superficial cancer, including multipolar electrocoagulation,[75] photodynamic therapy,[76] and argon plasma coagulation. A recent randomized controlled trial of radiofrequency ablation (RFA) in subjects who had dysplasia reported complete resolution of BE in over 75% of those treated with RFA, compared with 0% in control subjects.[77] A more complete discussion of ablative therapy is found in the article by Spechler and Davila in this issue.

EVIDENCE OF IMPROVED OUTCOMES
Impact Upon Mortality

The last and most crucial component of any effective screening strategy is that the implementation of the strategy in the target population reduces disease-specific mortality. Unfortunately, there has been no convincing data to show that screening for BE has made a meaningful impact on the mortality from ACE. All supportive data to this point have been plagued by lead-time bias, length bias, and selection bias, and no randomized controlled trials have been performed to compare screening and surveillance with no screening or surveillance.

Outcomes data from existing BE screening and surveillance programs have demonstrated that the tumors diagnosed through screening are at an earlier stage compared with those diagnosed via symptoms.[78] They also report short- and long-term (5-year) survival rates that are higher in the surveillance group than in the nonsurveillance group. In a retrospective cohort study of subjects who had distal ACE, Portale and colleagues[79] reported that those subjects who had BE had smaller tumors diagnosed at earlier stages, fewer metastases, and improved 5-year survival than those who did not have BE. They concluded that the ACE tumor characteristics were the same in both groups, but that the subjects who had BE had improved outcomes due to earlier detection of cancer.

Though these investigators argue that this is proof of the effectiveness of a screening and surveillance program, they do not address the inherent bias in these studies. Stage migration (the detection of cancer at earlier stages) is not well correlated with disease-specific mortality.[80] Length bias can be seen if the tumors found during screening examinations are slower growing, and inherently carry less morbidity and mortality than those that are unassociated with BE. Lead-time bias raises the possibility that screening and surveillance simply increase the time from known diagnosis to death instead of increasing true survival. These biases are likely alternative interpretations of the results seen in observational studies of the efficacy of screening programs. Graphical representations of length bias and lead-time bias are depicted in **Figs. 2** and **3**.

In one elegant demonstration of lead-time bias, Rubenstein and colleagues[81] showed that veterans who had an upper endoscopy (EGD) before diagnosis of ACE, and who were adherent to ACG guidelines for surveillance of BE, were diagnosed at earlier stages and initially demonstrated improved survival compared with subjects diagnosed with ACE who did not undergo EGD before diagnosis. However, 6 years postdiagnosis of ACE, there was no difference between the rate of survival

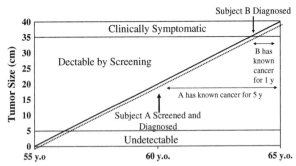

Fig. 2. Lead-time bias. Subject A and Subject B both develop ACE at age 55, time 0. Both are destined to live 10 years with their disease and die at age 65. Subject A undergoes screening and is diagnosed with ACE at age 60 when the cancer is asymptomatic. Subject B does not undergo screening and is diagnosed with cancer at age 64 when he presents with symptoms. Both die at age 65. Subject A lived 5 years after his diagnosis of cancer while Subject B only lived 1 year after his diagnosis. The screened patient Subject A has a prolonged time from diagnosis to death; however, his time from cancer development to death is identical to Subject B who does not undergo screening. X-axis: age of subject in years; Y-axis: length in cm of affected segment of esophagus.

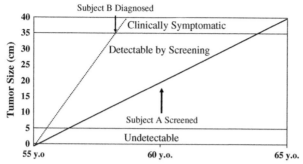

Fig. 3. Length bias. Subject A and Subject B both develop ACE at age 55, time 0. Subject A develops a slowly growing cancer. He is destined to live 10 years with his disease. Subject B has a highly aggressive cancer and is destined to live less than 5 years with his disease. Subject A undergoes screening and is diagnosed with ACE at age 60 when the cancer is at an early stage and is asymptomatic. He lives 5 years beyond his diagnosis. Subject B does not undergo screening and is diagnosed with cancer at age 58 when he presents with symptoms and an advanced-stage tumor. Subject A lives 5 years after his diagnosis of cancer while Subject B lives less than 1 year after his diagnosis. Screening appears to have prolonged the lifespan of Subject A; however, his tumor is inherently less aggressive and carries a better prognosis than the tumor of Subject B. X-axis: age of subject in years; Y-axis: length in cm of affected segment of esophagus.

among the two groups. Additionally, it has been shown that elevated mortality rates in subjects who had BE are rarely due to ACE, and that BE surveillance programs fail to make an impact upon ACE mortality.[21,82,83] These two issues suggest that we should be cautious in ascribing benefits to endoscopic surveillance programs, and that there may be overinterpretation of the perceived benefits gained from screening.

Evidence of Harm

Another problem with BE screening programs is that screening may not only fail to impact mortality, but may actually increase the likelihood of harm. The potential number of esophageal tumors detected via screening and surveillance programs has been calculated to be approximately equal to the potential number of serious endoscopic complications if a screening program is instituted for the entire United States adult population with GERD.[50] It has also been shown that a diagnosis of BE with or without dysplasia drastically increases insurance premiums in the United States.[84]

SUMMARY

After reviewing the body of evidence that describes the utility of currently practiced endoscopic screening programs for BE, one comes to the disappointing conclusion that screening patients who have chronic GERD to identify BE and thus decrease mortality from ACE is a flawed, costly, and ineffective process. What, then, should change in the study of these interrelated diseases that might make the difference between an effective screening program and an ineffective one?

Improved epidemiologic evidence regarding the risk factors for ACE could make a considerable impact on the utility of any screening program. A possible scenario would be to shift the focus away from BE as the primary premalignant lesion, and toward GERD as the only clinical syndrome leading to the premalignant lesion. Future research may focus on improving risk-stratification for patients who have GERD symptoms to increase the yield of screening endoscopy. For instance, does a 26-year-old, aerobically fit woman who has GERD symptoms of 5 years' duration warrant the same screening recommendation as a 67-year-old white man who has had GERD symptoms and prominent truncal obesity for 20 years? We may also make headway in identifying those patients without GERD and without BE who are destined to develop ACE so that they may be incorporated into the screening algorithm.

The scientific developments in identifying BE through advanced endoscopic techniques and molecular pathology provide promising avenues for improving screening. These techniques are not yet widely available and certainly increase the overall cost of the procedure. Also, it is not clear that more efficacious identification of nondysplastic BE will result in fewer deaths from cancer. If a more targeted population at risk can be isolated, the addition of these novel imaging and staining techniques may, however, prove to be cost-effective.

Lastly, it is imperative that studies be done to assess the outcomes of any future screening programs and the impact upon the mortality from esophageal adenocarcinoma. In its current state, a randomized controlled trial of a screening intervention would be difficult given the low rate of disease in the current target population. In the future, however, if a more defined target population is isolated, trials of screening interventions should be attempted to overcome the selection bias, length bias, and lead-time bias that is inherent to all observational studies of screening interventions. A significant benefit must be demonstrated to overcome the known potential harm to patients that comes with the diagnosis of BE.

REFERENCES

1. Raffle AE, Gray JAM. Screening: evidence and practice. Oxford, New York: Oxford University Press; 2007.
2. Wilson JMG, Jungner G. The principles and practice of screening for disease. Geneva, Switzerland: World Health Organization; 1968.
3. Sampliner RE. Updated guidelines for the diagnosis, surveillance, and therapy of Barrett's esophagus. Am J Gastroenterol 2002;97:1888–95.
4. Hirota WK, Zuckerman MJ, Adler DG, et al. ASGE guideline: the role of endoscopy in the surveillance of premalignant conditions of the upper GI tract. Gastrointest Endosc 2006;63:570–80.
5. Wang KK, Wongkeesong M, Buttar NS. American Gastroenterological Association technical review on the role of the gastroenterologist in the management of esophageal carcinoma. Gastroenterology 2005;128:1471–505.
6. Wang KK, Sampliner RE. Updated guidelines 2008 for the diagnosis, surveillance and therapy of Barrett's esophagus. Am J Gastroenterol 2008;103:788–97.
7. Lagergren J, Bergstrom R, Lindgren A, et al. Symptomatic gastroesophageal reflux as a risk factor for esophageal adenocarcinoma. N Engl J Med 1999;340:825–31.
8. Montgomery E, Bronner MP, Goldblum JR, et al. Reproducibility of the diagnosis of dysplasia in Barrett's esophagus: a reaffirmation. Hum Pathol 2001;32:368–78.
9. Shaheen N, Ransohoff DF. Gastroesophageal reflux, Barrett's esophagus, and esophageal cancer: scientific review. JAMA 2002;287:1972–81.
10. Birkmeyer JD, Siewers AE, Finlayson EVA, et al. Hospital volume and surgical mortality in the United States. N Engl J Med 2002;346:1128–37.
11. Corley DA, Levin TR, Habel LA, et al. Surveillance and survival in Barrett's adenocarcinomas: a population-based study. Gastroenterology 2002;122:633–40.

12. Edelstein ZR, Farrow DC, Bronner MP, et al. Central adiposity and risk of Barrett's esophagus. Gastroenterology 2007;133:403–11.
13. Ronkainen J, Aro P, Storskrubb T, et al. Prevalence of Barrett's esophagus in the general population: an endoscopic study. Gastroenterology 2005;129:1825–31.
14. Rubenstein JH, Inadomi JM, Brill JV, et al. Cost utility of screening for Barrett's esophagus with esophageal capsule endoscopy versus conventional upper endoscopy. Clin Gastroenterol Hepatol 2007;5:312–8.
15. Gerson L, Lin OS. Cost-benefit analysis of capsule endoscopy compared with standard upper endoscopy for the detection of Barrett's esophagus. Clin Gastroenterol Hepatol 2007;5:319–25.
16. Inadomi JM, Sampliner R, Lagergren J, et al. Screening and surveillance for Barrett esophagus in high-risk groups: a cost-utility analysis. Ann Intern Med 2003;138:176–86.
17. Gerson LB, Groeneveld PW, Triadafilopoulos G. Cost-effectiveness model of endoscopic screening and surveillance in patients with gastroesophageal reflux disease. Clin Gastroenterol Hepatol 2004;2:868–79.
18. Eckardt VF, Kanzler G, Bernhard G. Life expectancy and cancer risk in patients with Barrett's esophagus: a prospective controlled investigation. Am J Med 2001; 111:33–7.
19. Skacel M, Petras RE, Gramlich TL, et al. The diagnosis of low-grade dysplasia in Barrett's esophagus and its implications for disease progression. Am J Gastroenterol 2000;95:3383–7.
20. van der Burgh A, Dees J, Hop WC, et al. Oesophageal cancer is an uncommon cause of death in patients with Barrett's oesophagus. Gut 1996;39:5–8.
21. Macdonald CE, Wicks AC, Playford RJ. Final results from 10 year cohort of patients undergoing surveillance for Barrett's oesophagus: observational study. BMJ 2000;321:1252–5.
22. Cook MB, Wild CP, Everett SM, et al. Risk of mortality and cancer incidence in Barrett's esophagus. Cancer Epidemiol Biomarkers Prev 2007;16:2090–6.
23. O'Connor JB, Falk GW, Richter JE. The incidence of adenocarcinoma and dysplasia in Barrett's esophagus: report on the Cleveland Clinic Barrett's esophagus registry. Am J Gastroenterol 1999;94:2037–42.
24. Drewitz DJ, Sampliner RE, Garewal HS. The incidence of adenocarcinoma in Barrett's esophagus: a prospective study of 170 patients followed 4.8 years. Am J Gastroenterol 1997;92:212–5.
25. Abrams JA, Fields S, Lightdale CJ, et al. Racial and ethnic disparities in the prevalence of Barrett's esophagus among patients who undergo upper endoscopy. Clin Gastroenterol Hepatol 2008;6:30–4.
26. Stoltey J, Reeba H, Ullah N, et al. Does Barrett's oesophagus develop over time in patients with chronic gastro-oesophageal reflux disease? Aliment Pharmacol Ther 2007;25:83–91.
27. Veldhuyzen Van Zanten SJO, Thomson ABR, Barkun AN, et al. The prevalence of Barrett's oesophagus in a cohort of 1040 Canadian primary care patients with uninvestigated dyspepsia undergoing prompt endoscopy. Aliment Pharmacol Ther 2006;23:595–9.
28. Gerson LB, Edson R, Lavori PW, et al. Use of a simple symptom questionnaire to predict Barrett's esophagus in patients with symptoms of gastroesophageal reflux. Am J Gastroenterol 2001;96:2005–12.
29. Lieberman DA, Oehlke M, Helfand M. Risk factors for Barrett's esophagus in community-based practice. GORGE consortium (Gastroenterology Outcomes Research Group in Endoscopy). Am J Gastroenterol 1997;92:1293–7.

30. Smith KJ, O'Brien SM, Smithers BM, et al. Interactions among smoking, obesity, and symptoms of acid reflux in Barrett's esophagus. Cancer Epidemiol Biomarkers Prev 2005;14:2481–6.
31. Brandt MG, Darling GE, Miller L. Symptoms, acid exposure and motility in patients with Barrett's esophagus. Can J Surg 2004;47:47–51.
32. Johnson DA, Winters C, Spurling TJ, et al. Esophageal acid sensitivity in Barrett's esophagus. J Clin Gastroenterol 1987;9:23–7.
33. Eloubeidi MA, Provenzale D. Health-related quality of life and severity of symptoms in patients with Barrett's esophagus and gastroesophageal reflux disease patients without Barrett's esophagus. Am J Gastroenterol 2000;95:1881–7.
34. Skinner DB, Walther BC, Riddell RH, et al. Barrett's esophagus. Comparison of benign and malignant cases. Ann Surg 1983;198:554–65.
35. Paraf F, Flejou JF, Pignon JP, et al. Surgical pathology of adenocarcinoma arising in Barrett's esophagus. Analysis of 67 cases. Am J Surg Pathol 1995;19:183–91.
36. Rosenberg JC, Budev H, Edwards RC, et al. Analysis of adenocarcinoma in Barrett's esophagus utilizing a staging system. Cancer 1985;55:1353–60.
37. Rajendra S, Kutty K, Karim N. Ethnic differences in the prevalence of endoscopic esophagitis and Barrett's esophagus: the long and short of it all. Dig Dis Sci 2004; 49:237–42.
38. Oberg S, Wenner J, Johansson J, et al. Barrett esophagus: risk factors for progression to dysplasia and adenocarcinoma. Ann Surg 2005;242:49–54.
39. Corey KE, Schmitz SM, Shaheen NJ. Does a surgical antireflux procedure decrease the incidence of esophageal adenocarcinoma in Barrett's esophagus? A meta-analysis. Am J Gastroenterol 2003;98:2390–4.
40. El-Serag HB, Aguirre T, Kuebeler M, et al. The length of newly diagnosed Barrett's oesophagus and prior use of acid suppressive therapy. Aliment Pharmacol Ther 2004;19:1255–60.
41. El-Serag HB, Aguirre TV, Davis S, et al. Proton pump inhibitors are associated with reduced incidence of dysplasia in Barrett's esophagus. Am J Gastroenterol 2004;99:1877–83.
42. Kendall BJ, Macdonald GA, Hayward NK, et al. Leptin and the risk of Barrett's oesophagus. Gut 2008;57:448–54.
43. Gerson LB, Ullah N, Fass R, et al. Does body mass index differ between patients with Barrett's oesophagus and patients with chronic gastro-oesophageal reflux disease? Aliment Pharmacol Ther 2007;25:1079–86.
44. Stein DJ, El-Serag HB, Kuczynski J, et al. The association of body mass index with Barrett's oesophagus. Aliment Pharmacol Ther 2005;22:1005–10.
45. Veugelers PJ, Porter GA, Guernsey DL, et al. Obesity and lifestyle risk factors for gastroesophageal reflux disease, Barrett's esophagus and esophageal adenocarcinoma. Dis Esophagus 2006;19:321–38.
46. Frystyk CSEVSFHØ J. Circulating levels of free insulin-like growth factors in obese subjects: the impact of Type 2 diabetes. Diabetes Metab Res Rev 1999;15:314–32.
47. van Blankenstein M, Bohmer CJ, Hop WC. The incidence of adenocarcinoma in Barrett's esophagus in an institutionalized population. Eur J Gastroenterol Hepatol 2004;16:903–7.
48. Douglas KR, Oscar WC, Michael S, et al. Screening for Barrett's esophagus in colonoscopy patients with and without heartburn. Gastroenterology 2003;125: 1670–7.
49. Ward EM, Wolfsen HC, Achem SR, et al. Barrett's esophagus is common in older men and women undergoing screening colonoscopy regardless of reflux symptoms. Am J Gastroenterol 2006;101:12–7.

50. Dellon ES, Shaheen NJ. Does screening for Barrett's esophagus and adenocarcinoma of the esophagus prolong survival? J Clin Oncol 2005;23:4478–82.
51. Solaymani-Dodaran M, Logan RFA, West J, et al. Mortality associated with Barrett's esophagus and gastroesophageal reflux disease diagnoses—a population-based cohort study. Am J Gastroenterol 2005;100:2616–21.
52. Hage M, Siersema PD, van Dekken H, et al. Oesophageal cancer incidence and mortality in patients with long-segment Barrett's oesophagus after a mean follow-up of 12.7 years. Scand J Gastroenterol 2004;39:1175–9.
53. Solaymani-Dodaran M, Logan RF, West J, et al. Risk of oesophageal cancer in Barrett's oesophagus and gastro-oesophageal reflux. Gut 2004;53:1070–4.
54. Basu KK, Pick B, de Caestecker JS. Audit of a Barrett's epithelium surveillance database. Eur J Gastroenterol Hepatol 2004;16:171–5.
55. Gareth SD, Sushovan G, Katherine LK, et al. Preoperative prevalence of Barrett's esophagus in esophageal adenocarcinoma: a systematic review. Gastroenterology 2002;122:26–33.
56. Lassen A, Hallas J, de Muckadell OBS. Esophagitis: incidence and risk of esophageal adenocarcinoma—a population-based cohort study. Am J Gastroenterol 2006;101:1193–9.
57. Theisen J, Stein HJ, Dittler HJ, et al. Preoperative chemotherapy unmasks underlying Barrett's mucosa in patients with adenocarcinoma of the distal esophagus. Surg Endosc 2002;16:671–3.
58. Eloubeidi MA, Provenzale D. Does this patient have Barrett's esophagus? The utility of predicting Barrett's esophagus at the index endoscopy. Am J Gastroenterol 1999;94:937–43.
59. Harrison R, Perry I, Haddadin W, et al. Detection of intestinal metaplasia in Barrett's esophagus: an observational comparator study suggests the need for a minimum of eight biopsies. Am J Gastroenterol 2007;102:1154–61.
60. Iascone C, DeMeester TR, Little AG, et al. Barrett's esophagus: functional assessment, proposed pathogenesis, and surgical therapy. Arch Surg 1983;118:543–59.
61. Loughney T, Maydonovitch CL, Wong RK. Esophageal manometry and ambulatory 24-hour pH monitoring in patients with short and long segment Barrett's esophagus. Am J Gastroenterol 1998;93:916–9.
62. Sharma P, Dent J, Armstrong D, et al. The development and validation of an endoscopic grading system for Barrett's esophagus: the prague C&M criteria. Gastroenterology 2006;131:1392–9.
63. Sharma P, Topalovski M, Mayo MS, et al. Methylene blue chromoendoscopy for detection of short-segment Barrett's esophagus. Gastrointest Endosc 2001;54:289–93.
64. Reid BJ, Blount PL, Feng Z, et al. Optimizing endoscopic biopsy detection of early cancers in Barrett's high-grade dysplasia. Am J Gastroenterol 2000;95:3089–96.
65. MacNeil-Covin L, Casson AG, Malatjalian D, et al. A survey of Canadian gastroenterologists about the management of Barrett's esophagus. Can J Gastroenterol 2003;17:313–7.
66. Amamra N, Touzet S, Colin C, et al. Current practice compared with the international guidelines: endoscopic surveillance of Barrett's esophagus. J Eval Clin Pract 2007;13:789–94.
67. Sarbia M, Donner A, Franke C, et al. Distinction between intestinal metaplasia in the cardia and in Barrett's esophagus: the role of histology and immunohistochemistry. Hum Pathol 2004;35:371–6.

68. Ormsby AH, Petras RE, Henricks WH, et al. Observer variation in the diagnosis of superficial oesophageal adenocarcinoma. Gut 2002;51:671–6.

69. Lenglinger J, Ringhofer C, Eisler M, et al. Histopathology of columnar-lined esophagus in patients with gastroesophageal reflux disease. Wien Klin Wochenschr 2007;119:405–11.

70. Canto MI, Setrakian S, Willis J, et al. Methylene blue-directed biopsies improve detection of intestinal metaplasia and dysplasia in Barrett's esophagus. Gastrointest Endosc 2000;51:560–8.

71. Sharma P, Weston AP, Topalovski M, et al. Magnification chromoendoscopy for the detection of intestinal metaplasia and dysplasia in Barrett's oesophagus. Gut 2003;52:24–7.

72. Sharma P, Bansal A, Mathur S, et al. The utility of a novel narrow band imaging endoscopy system in patients with Barrett's esophagus. Gastrointest Endosc 2006;64:167–75.

73. Eliakim R, Sharma VK, Yassin K, et al. A prospective study of the diagnostic accuracy of PillCam ESO esophageal capsule endoscopy versus conventional upper endoscopy in patients with chronic gastroesophageal reflux diseases. J Clin Gastroenterol 2005;39:572–8.

74. Saeian K, Staff DM, Vasilopoulos S, et al. Unsedated transnasal endoscopy accurately detects Barrett's metaplasia and dysplasia. Gastrointest Endosc 2002;56: 472–8.

75. Dulai GS, Jensen DM, Cortina G, et al. Randomized trial of argon plasma coagulation versus multipolar electrocoagulation for ablation of Barrett's esophagus. Gastrointest Endosc 2005;61:232–40.

76. Overholt BF, Lightdale CJ, Wang KK, et al. Photodynamic therapy with porfimer sodium for ablation of high-grade dysplasia in Barrett's esophagus: international, partially blinded, randomized phase III trial. Gastrointest Endosc 2005;62: 488–98.

77. Shaheen N, Sharma P, Overholt BF, et al. A randomized, multicenter, sham-controlled trial of radiofrequency ablation (RFA) for subjects with Barrett's esophagus (BE) containing dysplasia: interim results of the AIM Dysplasia Trial. Presented at the 109th annual meeting of the AGA Institute during Digestive Disease Week. May 18–22, 2008. San Diego, CA: American Gastroenterological Association Institute; 2008, vol. 134. p. P51.

78. Aldulaimi DM, Cox M, Nwokolo CU, et al. Barrett's surveillance is worthwhile and detects curable cancers. A prospective cohort study addressing cancer incidence, treatment outcome and survival. Eur J Gastroenterol Hepatol 2005;17: 943–50.

79. Portale G, Peters JH, Hagen JA, et al. Comparison of the clinical and histological characteristics and survival of distal esophageal-gastroesophageal junction adenocarcinoma in patients with and without Barrett mucosa. Arch Surg 2005; 140:570–5.

80. Welch HG, Schwartz LM, Woloshin S. Are increasing 5-year survival rates evidence of success against cancer? JAMA 2000;283:2975–8.

81. Rubenstein JH, Sonnenberg A, Davis J, et al. Effect of a prior endoscopy on outcomes of esophageal adenocarcinoma among United States veterans. Gastrointest Endosc 2008.

82. Quera R, O'Sullivan K, Quigley EM. Surveillance in Barrett's Oesophagus: will a strategy focused on a high-risk group reduce mortality from oesophageal adenocarcinoma? Endoscopy 2006;162–9.

83. Chang LC, Oelschlager BK, Quiroga E, et al. Long-term outcome of esophagec-tomy for high-grade dysplasia or cancer found during surveillance for Barrett's esophagus. J Gastrointest Surg 2006;10:341–6.
84. Shaheen NJ, Dulai GS, Ascher B, et al. Effect of a new diagnosis of Barrett's esophagus on insurance status. Am J Gastroenterol 2005;100:577–80.

Role of Obesity in Barrett's Esophagus and Cancer

Liam Murray, MD[a],*, Yvonne Romero, MD[b]

KEYWORDS

- Reflux esophagitis • Barrett's esophagus
- Esophageal adenocarcinoma • Obesity • Adiposity

The incidence of esophageal adenocarcinoma (EAC) has increased dramatically in the western world over the last 30 years,[1] and although the trends in the diagnosis of Barrett's esophagus (BE) are more difficult to interpret because of substantial increases in the use of endoscopy over this period and improvement in physician recognition,[2] it remains possible that there has been some increase in the incidence of BE and gastroesophageal reflux disease (GERD) in recent years.[3] The contemporaneous increase in obesity in the western world has focused interest on whether obesity is a risk factor for EAC and its precursors, whereas the failure of overall obesity to explain the basic patterns of EAC distribution (eg, the sex differences and differences between ethnic groups[1]) has led to a focus on body fat distribution and abdominal obesity. Much interest has also been shown in the mechanisms whereby overweight or obesity may increase risk of this disease spectrum. This article reviews current evidence for the role that overweight/obesity and body fat distribution have in development of the esophagitis-metaplasia-dysplasia-adenocarcinoma sequence. Particular attention is paid to the stage at which adiposity may act to influence the risk of EAC, because this determines the importance of weight control and weight loss at each stage in the disease spectrum for the prevention of EAC.

IS ADIPOSITY A RISK FACTOR FOR REFLUX SYMPTOMS AND EROSIVE REFLUX ESOPHAGITIS, AND DO THE RELATIONSHIPS DIFFER FOR OVERALL AND ABDOMINAL OBESITY?

A large body of evidence has examined the relationship between adiposity and GERD symptoms (heartburn and acid regurgitation) and erosive esophagitis. In a meta-analysis of studies examining the association between body mass index (BMI) and reflux symptoms, Hampel and colleagues[4] identified nine robust cross-sectional studies that

[a] Centre for Public Health, The Queen's University of Belfast, Mulhouse Building, Grosvenor Road, Belfast B12 6BJ, UK
[b] Division of Gastroenterology and Hepatology, Departments of Medicine and Otorhinolaryngology, Mayo Clinic College of Medicine, 200 First Street SW, Rochester, MN 55905, USA
* Corresponding author.
E-mail address: murray@qub.ac.uk (L. Murray).

Surg Oncol Clin N Am 18 (2009) 439–452
doi:10.1016/j.soc.2009.03.010
1055-3207/09/$ – see front matter © 2009 Elsevier Inc. All rights reserved.

included a total of 7373 subjects with symptoms and 55,603 without symptoms. All of the studies showed positive relationships between being overweight or obese and the presence of GERD symptoms; the pooled odds ratios (ORs) with 95% confidence intervals (95% CI) for overweight and obesity were 1.43 (1.16 to 1.78) and 1.94 (1.16 to 1.77), respectively. Only one of these studies reported findings separately for men and women, and relationships were somewhat stronger in women. The meta-analysis also included seven studies (4668 cases and 23,899 controls) that examined the association between BMI and erosive reflux esophagitis. All but one of these studies also showed positive associations; the pooled OR (95% CI) for overweight/obese (combined) was 1.76 (1.16 to 2.68), with stronger associations seen in obese men when compared with obese women. This meta-analysis showed that being overweight and obese, as measured by BMI, was associated with GERD symptoms and erosive esophagitis, but a higher BMI, even within the normal range, was also positively associated with GERD symptoms.[5] More recent population-based studies have confirmed the association between being overweight or obese and GERD symptoms.[6,7]

Few studies have examined the relationship between GERD symptoms and measures of adiposity other than BMI, which is a measure of overall adiposity and therefore provides no information on the distribution of body fat. Among 80,000 members of the Kaiser Permanente Health Plan in San Francisco and Oakland, California, Corley and colleagues[8] showed that increased abdominal adiposity (measured by abdominal diameter) was associated with GERD symptoms even after adjustment for BMI (and other potential confounders) in whites but not in blacks or Asians. Adjusted ORs for the highest compared with lowest category of abdominal diameter were 1.85 (1.55 to 2.21), 0.95 (0.61 to 1.48), and 0.64 (0.18 to 2.30) for whites, blacks, and Asians respectively, with similar findings in white men and women. BMI was also associated with symptoms in this study; this association was attenuated somewhat by adjustment for abdominal diameter, suggesting that at least part of the relationship between BMI and GERD symptoms is mediated by abdominal obesity. In the Nurses' Health Study, a high waist-hip ratio (WHR) was also associated with GERD symptoms (OR [95% CI] for the highest quintile versus lowest quintile of WHR, 1.88 [1.45 to 2.45]), but in contrast to the Kaiser Permanente study, this association was blunted by adjustment for BMI.[5]

Two recently published studies performed in patients undergoing endoscopy in Korean medical centers have shown strong associations between abdominal adiposity and erosive reflux esophagitis. In one of these studies,[9] the OR (95% CI) for esophagitis in subjects with abdominal obesity (defined as a waist circumference ≥80 cm in women and ≥90 cm in men) was 2.3 (1.6 to 3.1), and this relationship was independent of BMI. In the second study,[10] the ORs for esophagitis in subjects with a WHR greater than 1 or 0.8 to 1 compared with less than 0.8 were 4.1 and 2.3, respectively. Although these results may not be generalizable to non-Asian populations, they provide evidence that abdominal obesity may be more important in the development of erosive esophagitis than overall obesity.

Strong evidence suggests that overall obesity is a risk factor for both GERD symptoms and erosive reflux esophagitis, with marginal evidence of a stronger association in men than women. Abdominal obesity has been shown to be a risk factor for GERD symptoms in whites, but this may not be true in blacks and Asians, and it is unclear whether abdominal obesity is a stronger risk factor for GERD than overall obesity. Recent evidence from Asian populations suggests that abdominal obesity rather than overall obesity increases esophagitis risk.

DOES WEIGHT LOSS IN OBESE OR OVERWEIGHT PATIENTS IMPROVE SYMPTOMS OF GASTROESOPHAGEAL REFLUX DISEASE OR EROSIVE ESOPHAGITIS OR PREVENT THE DEVELOPMENT OF BARRETT'S ESOPHAGUS?

Although there is a paucity of data with which to address this question and although not all studies are in agreement,[11] weight loss in obese or overweight patients appears to improve GERD symptoms,[12,13] reduce acid reflux into the esophagus,[14] and improve histologic and clinical esophagitis.[15] Loss of visceral/abdominal fat may be particularly important in reducing reflux.[14] The question of whether weight loss in patients with esophagitis will reduce the risk of developing BE has not yet been addressed.

IS ADIPOSITY A RISK FACTOR FOR BARRETT'S ESOPHAGUS, AND DO THE RELATIONSHIPS DIFFER FOR OVERALL AND ABDOMINAL OBESITY?

To date, few studies have examined the relationship between BMI and BE. In a small retrospective cross-sectional study of patients undergoing endoscopy within the Southern Arizona Veteran's Affairs Healthcare System,[16] 65 patients with BE were compared with 385 patients without BE. Being overweight or obese was associated with the risk of BE; the ORs (95% CI) for overweight and obese patients compared with normal weight patients were 2.43 (1.12 to 5.31) and 2.46 (1.11 to 5.44), respectively. Bu and colleagues[17] showed similar findings in another study of endoscopy patients; however, the control groups in these studies do not represent the normal population and may therefore generate misleading results. Cook and colleagues[18] undertook a meta-analysis of studies comparing BMI in BE cases with population controls. Only three studies were identified,[19–21] which gave a pooled OR (95% CI) per unit increase in BMI of 1.02 (1.01 to 1.04). This finding was a substantially more modest increase in risk than that seen in the descriptive cohort reports of endoscopy patients.

A recently published study has examined the relationships between overall and abdominal adiposity measured by WHR and BE risk.[22] In this case-control study (which included 211 population controls), a high WHR was associated (after adjustment for confounders and BMI) with an substantially increased risk of BE, whether BE was defined as specialized intestinal metaplasia (SIM) positive (197 cases), SIM positive with a visible Barrett's segment (97 cases), or SIM positive with a visible long segment BE (54 cases). ORs (95% CI) for the three groups were 1.9 (1.1 to 3.2), 2.9 (1.5 to 5.7), and 4.1 (1.7 to 10.0), respectively. Corresponding ORs (95% CI) adjusted for confounders and WHR for overall obesity (defined as BMI ≥30) were 2.0 (1.1 to 3.5), 1.0 (0.5 to 2.0), and 1.2 (0.5 to 3.0), respectively. Abdominal adiposity was a strong risk factor for BE surviving adjustment for BMI, whereas, in contrast, the weaker association with BMI was attenuated by adjustment for the WHR ratio. Furthermore, the associations with WHR were strengthened rather than attenuated by adjustment for reflux symptoms, suggesting that central adiposity may exert its effect on BE risk by mechanisms that are independent of perception of reflux.

Similar results were obtained in a case-control study of 320 incident BE cases and 317 population controls undertaken within the Kaiser Permanente Northern California population.[23] In that study, abdominal circumference between 80 cm (32 inches) and 89 cm (35 inches) was related to BE risk; the OR (95% CI) adjusted for BMI was 2.24 (1.21 to 4.15). There was no increase in the risk of BE in cases with larger waist sizes ranging from 90 to greater than 130 cm, and there was no evidence of a dose-response curve (ie, the higher the waist circumference the higher the risk of BE). In contrast, adiposity as judged by BMI was not associated with the risk of BE. Abdominal circumference was associated with GERD symptoms, and some attenuation of the association between waist circumference and BE was seen on adjustment for these symptoms; statistical significance was lost, but the OR (95% CI) remained elevated (1.78 [0.86 to 3.66]).

The findings of these two studies are supported by those of a small retrospective study of 36 BE patients and 93 controls (BE-negative endoscopy cases) in whom visceral and subcutaneous adipose tissue was measured from abdominal CT scans taken within 1 year of endoscopy. Visceral adipose tissue was 1.5 fold greater in cases than in controls (183 versus 115 cm,^{2} P <.001). Differences were also seen between cases and controls for subcutaneous adipose tissue, but these were less marked (248 versus 200 cm^2), and in a multivariate model, visceral adipose tissue but not BMI was significantly associated with BE.

Data from these studies indicate that the distribution of body fat may be important in determining the risk of BE, suggesting that abdominal obesity appears to be a stronger risk factor than overall obesity. The data also indicate that at least part of the relationship between abdominal obesity and BE is mediated by mechanisms other than GERD symptoms.

IS THE INCREASED RISK OF BARRETT'S ESOPHAGUS IN OBESE OR OVERWEIGHT INDIVIDUALS INDEPENDENT OF THE INCREASE IN RISK OF ESOPHAGITIS?

Cook and colleagues[18] have recently explored whether adiposity presents an additional risk for BE over and above that associated with GERD/GERD symptoms. A stronger association between BE and adiposity would indicate that adiposity could predict which GERD patients will develop BE. Consequently, screening and surveillance of overweight GERD patients might facilitate the early detection of BE, and weight reduction in such patients might reduce the risk of BE and possibly EAC. Cook explored this question by undertaking a meta-analysis of observational studies in which BE cases were compared with GERD controls (with or without confirmed esophagitis) or normal population controls. BMI was used as the proxy of adiposity in these studies. Although BMI was positively associated with BE when the comparison group was population controls, this was not true when BE cases were compared with GERD controls (no difference between studies with confirmed esophagitis controls and those in whom esophagitis was not confirmed). It was concluded that increasing adiposity presents no additional risk for BE beyond increasing the risk of GERD/GERD symptoms alone. A further study, which was not included in Cook's meta-analysis (published after the literature search), agreed with the findings of the meta-analysis. The BMI in 165 patients diagnosed with BE was not different from that in 586 patients with endoscopically proven esophagitis or gastroesophageal reflux proven by 24-hour pH monitoring.[24] The recent case-control study from the Kaiser Permanente Northern California population[23] also included a GERD symptom control group. In that study, although waist circumference and the waist/thigh ratio were associated with BE in a comparison with population controls, the relationship between BE and these measures of abdominal adiposity were weaker and not statistically significant when the comparison group was the GERD controls. It is possible that general or abdominal adiposity increases the risk of BE by principally increasing the risk of GERD/GERD symptoms.

IS ADIPOSITY A RISK FACTOR FOR ESOPHAGEAL ADENOCARCINOMA, AND DO THE RELATIONSHIPS DIFFER FOR OVERALL AND ABDOMINAL OBESITY?

Adiposity is a risk factor for EAC.[19,25,26] Estimates of the degree of association between obesity and EAC differ between reports most likely because of differences in study design. Some studies estimated obesity based on subject recall of their height and weight in youth or years prior to the diagnosis of cancer, whereas other studies had access to objective measurements collected in the past. In contrast, obesity is not a risk factor for squamous cell carcinoma of the esophagus.[25–27]

A meta-analysis of 14 observational studies (12 case-control and 2 cohort studies)[28] showed an association between being overweight or obese and EAC risk; pooled ORs (95% CI) for the two groups were 1.9 (1.5 to 2.4) and 2.4 (2.0 to 2.8), respectively, with a slightly stronger association in men than women. Abnet and colleagues[29] identified an association between BMI and EAC in a large cohort study. The risk of EAC in a NIH-AARP Diet and Health Study cohort (which included almost 500,000 participants) increased with increasing baseline BMI (based on self-reported height and weight), and the (adjusted) hazard ratio for participants with a BMI in the highest category ($\geq$ 35) when compared with participants with a normal BMI was 2.27 (1.44 to 3.59). In a meta-analysis of prospective studies examining the association between BMI and the incidence of 20 different types of cancer, the strongest association in men was for EAC; it was the third strongest association in women.[30]

Corley and colleagues[27] examined the associations between abdominal and overall obesity (BMI) and EAC risk in a nested case-control study within the Multiphasic Health Check-up cohort in Northern California. The abdominal diameter at baseline (between 1965 and 1969 inclusively) was compared between 101 participants who subsequently developed EAC and matched controls who did not develop this cancer. A larger abdominal diameter was associated with EAC; the OR (95% CI) for the highest compared with lowest quartile was 3.47 (1.29 to 9.33). BMI was also associated with EAC risk; the OR (95% CI) for a BMI of 30 or greater compared with normal was 3.17 (1.43 to 7.04). The relationship between abdominal diameter and EAC risk was strengthened on adjustment for BMI and was unaltered by adjustment for GERD symptoms. Abdominal diameter was not associated with cardiac adenocarcinoma or squamous cell carcinoma. These findings suggest that both overall adiposity and abdominal adiposity may independently increase the risk of EAC, and that abdominal adiposity may increase EAC risk by a mechanism unrelated to the induction of GERD symptoms. The results of this study are supported by a small study that examined 30 incident cases of adenocarcinoma of the gastric cardia and lower third of the esophagus (combined) within an Australian cohort study.[31] This study showed a positive association with both BMI and abdominal circumference. The hazard ratio (95% CI) for a BMI of 30 or greater compared with a BMI of less than 25 was 3.7 (1.1 to 12.4) and the hazard ratio per 10 cm increase in abdominal circumference, 1.46 (1.05 to 2.04). The hazard ratio (95%) per 10 kg increase in fat-free mass (measured by bioelectrical impedance) was also increased in this study (2.06 [1.15 to 3.68]).

A study using the resources of the Rochester Epidemiology Project, a population-based study reviewing the records of all persons diagnosed with EAC (N = 29) from 1971 to 2000 with records dating back in some cases to their birth, did not demonstrate an association between BMI and EAC.[32] Cases were matched with randomly selected population controls of like age ($\pm$1 year) and sex who were seen by a local provider in the same year ($\pm$1 year) that the case was diagnosed. Several height and weight measurements were available over each person's lifetime. A history of GERD was significantly associated with EAC (OR [95% CI], 5.5 [1.2 to 24.8]). Neither a BMI greater than 30 nor a maximal lifetime BMI greater than 30 were associated with EAC (OR [95% CI], 1.7 [0.4 to 7.0] and 1.3 [0.6 to 3.0]), respectively; however, this was a small study.

Overall, emerging data suggest that being overweight or obese is associated with an increased risk of EAC, and that abdominal adiposity is at least as important a risk factor as is general adiposity. What is less clear is at what stage in the disease process adiposity acts to increase EAC risk. The association between obesity early in life and subsequent EAC risk[19,25] together with the data suggesting that adiposity increases BE risk by principally increasing the risk of esophagitis[18] suggest that adiposity may act early in the disease process. Most studies that have examined the relationship between obesity and EAC risk have shown it to be independent of reflux symptoms.[19,22,25,27] Although this finding may reflect the insensitivity of symptom-based measures of assessing gastroesophageal reflux, obesity could also act to increase EAC risk by mechanisms that are unrelated to reflux, such as via insulin-like growth factors, and these mechanisms may operate later in the disease process. Alternatively, obesity-induced reflux may continue to occur during the later stages of the disease process (eg, after the development of the less acid-sensitive Barrett's epithelium) and be an important determinant of progression from BE to EAC.

Family studies also show obesity to be an important risk factor in BE and EAC. In a cohort study comparing the risk factors for EAC and adenocarcinoma of the gastric cardia in relatives with a family history of BE, EAC, or adenocarcinoma of the gastric cardia versus those who lacked this family history, after adjusting for confounders, obesity was associated with EAC and adenocarcinoma of the gastric cardia diagnosed at an early age (personal communication, A. Chak, March 2009). In another family study, first-degree relatives of BE or EAC probands were obese more often than endoscopy controls, although the results were not statistically significant; 44% of symptomatic relatives were obese versus 39% of symptomatic controls and 22% of asymptomatic relatives versus 19% of controls (personal communication, Y. Romero, March 2009). Aggregation of GERD symptoms in families[33,34] could be due to shared or learned environmental behaviors such as diet, exercise, or lack thereof, or could be due to a genetic propensity for obesity or a susceptibility to esophageal damage in response to reflux. Although the role of family history in BE and EAC is actively under investigation, it appears that obesity has role in familial aggregation of GERD symptoms, BE, and EAC.

IS OBESITY ASSOCIATED WITH THE PROGRESSION FROM BARRETT'S ESOPHAGUS TO ESOPHAGEAL ADENOCARCINOMA, AND DOES THIS DIFFER FOR OVERALL AND ABDOMINAL OBESITY?

Studies that have compared measures of adiposity between EAC cases and BE controls can provide some insight into this question. One such study has been undertaken within the Netherlands.[35] In this hospital-based, case-control study, EAC cases were more likely than BE controls to have been overweight (BMI ≥25) at age 20 and 10 years before diagnosis; the adjusted ORs (95% CI) were 2.6 (1.2 to 5.5) and 1.8 (1.1 to 3.3), respectively. The stronger association at age 20 years than at 10 years before diagnosis also points to the importance of adiposity early in life, presumably before the development of BE. Data from the Irish FINBAR case-control study of EAC and BE showed that EAC cases were more likely to be overweight or obese 5 years before diagnosis than age- and sex-matched BE controls; ORs (95% CI) were 1.70 (1.03 to 2.79) and 3.32 (1.84 to 6.00), respectively (Murray L, unpublished data, 2008).

Further evidence of whether adiposity influences EAC risk in BE patients could be provided by examination of the intermediate stages in the progression to cancer (eg, dysplasia) or other markers for progression. One small study of 140 dysplasia-free BE patients has prospectively explored factors associated with the progression to low-grade dysplasia (mean follow-up period, 5.8 years).[36] Forty-four patients (31.4%) progressed to low-grade dysplasia and seven to high-grade dysplasia or

EAC. BMI was not associated with the development of either low-grade dysplasia or high-grade dysplasia/EAC; however, this was a small study with limited power to detect associations between BMI and disease progression. Data from a cross-sectional study within the Seattle Barrett's Esophagus Project[37] have shown that the WHR is associated with a range of potential markers for progression to EAC (eg, 4N and aneuploidy on flow cytometry and 17p and 9p loss of heterozygosity). The OR for aneuploidy comparing the highest to lowest quartile of WHR was 4.3 (1.2 to 15.6) and for 17p loss of heterozygosity, 3.9 (1.3 to 11.4). In contrast, BMI, a measure of general adiposity, was not associated with these markers; the OR (95% CI) for aneuploidy, obese subjects (BMI $\geq$30) when compared with normal weight subjects (BMI <25) was 0.9 (0.3 to 2.9) and for 17p loss of heterozygosity, 0.9 (0.3 to 2.3). These data suggest that abdominal adiposity may be more important in determining future EAC risk than overall adiposity, but this was not a prospective study, the participants were in general high-risk BE patients, and the outcomes examined were markers associated with progression to cancer rather than cancer itself.

There is a lack of appropriately designed studies to investigate whether being overweight or obese increases the risk of progression from BE to EAC. Nevertheless, this question is fundamental to the management of BE patients. Further studies examining other biomarkers of progression (eg, telomere length,[38] measures of oxidative DNA damage,[39] or perhaps DNA methylation patterns[40,41]) as outcomes may be useful, but this question can only be adequately addressed by undertaking large (probably multicenter) prospective studies of BE patients with detailed anthropometric measurements taken at baseline and with sufficient length of follow-up to enable EAC or high-grade dysplasia to be examined as an outcome.

CAN WEIGHT LOSS PREVENT DISEASE PROGRESSION IN PATIENTS WITH BARRETT'S ESOPHAGUS?

Only one intervention study has investigated whether weight loss in BE patients, as part of a dietary intervention that included increased fruit and vegetable and decreased fat intake, affects biomarkers of cellular proliferation in Barrett's epithelium.[42] This study randomized 93 patients to receive the diet/weight loss intervention or usual diet. The intervention group successfully lost weight (mean 3.6 kg loss at 18 months and 2.5 kg at 36 months); fruit and vegetable intake also increased. No difference was seen between the two groups in changes from baseline in the flow cytometric markers of cellular proliferation, percent Ki67-positive proliferating diploid G_1 cells, or percent total Ki67-positive proliferating cells, or in the presence of more than 6% of cells in the 4N fraction of the cell cycle. In this small study the dietary/weight loss changes may not have been of sufficient magnitude and duration to observe changes in the markers, or the intervention may have affected earlier stages in the neoplastic process than those assessed by the markers. Further trials of weight loss in BE with alternative markers of progression may help shed light on this area, but only large trials with EAC or high-grade dysplasia as the outcome can conclusively determine whether weight loss in BE patients can reduce cancer risk. Such studies may be so expensive and difficult to undertake that they will not be considered until reliable data are provided from large cohort studies documenting that obesity is associated with progression from BE to EAC.

An extremely small case series described the outcomes of five morbidly obese, long segment, biopsy-proven Barrett's esophagus patients who underwent Roux-en-Y gastrojejunostomy.[43] The BMI changed from 43 kg/m^2 to 33 kg/m^2, and all patients reported subjective improvement in reflux symptoms. Preoperatively, the mean BE length was 6 ± 2 cm; two patients had low-grade dysplasia and one indeterminate dysplasia. At their postoperative surveillance endoscopy performed at least 1 year after surgery, the length of the BE segment had either decreased (in two patients) or completely disappeared (in two patients) for a mean length 2 ± 1 cm, and only one patient had dysplasia. In this small case series, Roux-en-Y gastrojejunostomy resulted in complete or partial regression of BE in four of five patients with improvement in reflux symptoms in all.

POTENTIAL MECHANISMS OF ACTION FOR RELATIONSHIP BETWEEN OBESITY AND BARRETT'S ESOPHAGUS/ESOPHAGEAL ADENOCARCINOMA (OR REFLUX DISEASE IN GENERAL)

Obesity may contribute to gastroesophageal reflux through several anatomic and physiologic mechanisms (eg, increased intra-abdominal pressure and development of hiatus hernia,[44] increased intragastric pressure and gastroesophageal sphincter gradient,[45] slower esophageal transit times,[46] and increased transient relaxations of the lower esophageal sphincter[47]). Few studies have distinguished between overall obesity and abdominal obesity, but one recent study showed a similar, albeit weak, positive correlation between the BMI and waist circumference and intragastric pressure.[48] Clearly, promotion of gastroesophageal reflux is an important mechanism whereby overweight or obesity increases the risk of EAC or BE, but because at least part of the association between obesity and EAC appears to be independent of reflux, alternative mechanisms exist. A potential role for reflux-independent mechanisms is also likely given that obesity increases the risk of a variety of cancers unrelated to gastroesophageal reflux.

Adipose tissue is now regarded as the largest endocrine organ of the body. As well as being a major site for the metabolism of sex steroids and glucocorticoids, adipose tissue expresses and secretes a range of metabolically active factors (adipokines), including free fatty acids, interleukin (IL)-6, IL-8, tumor necrosis factor-α, leptin, adiponectin, plasminogen activator inhibitor-1, and resistin,[49] and visceral fat is more metabolically active than subcutaneous fat.[50] In general, these adipokines are proinflammatory, promote insulin resistance, and have a central role in the development of atherosclerosis. The induction of insulin resistance may also be important to cancer development. Chronically high insulin levels may promote proliferation and inhibit apoptosis via insulin receptors or alter the insulin-like growth factor (IGF) axis, resulting in reduced IGF-binding proteins (IGFBP) and higher levels of free IGF-1. Altered IGFBP-3 and IGF-1 levels have been associated with the development of several cancers, including breast, colorectal, and prostate cancer.[51–55] Gene expression studies in animals[56] and humans[57,58] indicate a potential role for the IGF axis in the progression of BE to EAC, and a recently reported prospective study has shown an association between low IGFBP-3 levels and aneuploidy risk in BE patients.[59] Polymorphism of the IGFBP-3 gene was also associated with aneuploidy risk. These studies indicate that the IGF axis may have a role in mediating the association between obesity and EAC, and further investigation of this pathway is warranted.

Adiponectin, an important adipokine, is strongly inversely associated with central and overall obesity and with insulin resistance.[60] Low levels of adiponectin have been associated with breast,[61] endometrial,[62,63] colorectal,[64] and other cancers, and these associations appear to be largely independent of other obesity-related risk factors such as endogenous insulin concentration, IGF-binding proteins, or hormonal status.[60] Evidence is accumulating that adiponectin is an important regulator of cell proliferation; it can induce apoptosis, decrease the expression of cyclin

D1 and inhibit cell-cycle progression, and inhibit growth factors.[60] Adiponectin also has anti-inflammatory effects, including the induction of anti-inflammatory cytokines.[65] There are several ways in which adiponectin may influence the development of cancers in general or EAC in particular. Few studies have examined the role of adiponectin in relation to the development of BE or EAC. Adiponectin receptors were found to be down-regulated in the Barrett's mucosa of 15 obese BE patients when compared with normal squamous esophageal mucosa from the same patients.[66] The same group also showed an increase in the expression of the pro-apoptotic protein Bax, a decrease in expression of the anti-apoptotic protein Bcl-2, and a dose-dependent increase in apoptosis after incubation of an EAC cell line with adiponectin. A pilot epidemiologic study showed no association between adiponectin levels in 51 BE patients when compared with 67 controls,[67] but this was a small study that did not investigate whether adiponectin has a role in the progression of BE to EAC. These findings need to be re-examined in other BE case-control studies, and prospective investigations of the role that adiponectin may have in the progression of BE to EAC are required.

Leptin is another adipokine secreted by adipocytes and gastric chief cells that may have a role in the development of BE and EAC. Circulating leptin levels are closely positively correlated with total body fat and are higher in women than men, even after allowing for differences in fat mass.[68] Leptin has been shown to stimulate cell proliferation and inhibit apoptosis in in vitro studies, including studies of EAC cell lines,[69,70] and leptin receptors are expressed in the adult esophagus.[71] Some epidemiologic studies show positive associations between leptin levels and breast, colorectal, and prostate cancer, although the data are somewhat inconsistent.[72–74] A recent epidemiologic study has examined the relationship between serum leptin concentration and BE risk.[67] In this population-based, case-control study, leptin levels were strongly associated with the risk of BE in men but not women. In another study undertaken in an endoscopy population from a veteran's administration medical center in New York, gastric but not serum leptin levels were positively associated with BE. Further study of the relationship between leptin and BE/EAC is warranted.

Ghrelin is a peptide produced mainly in the fundus of the stomach that, among other functions, stimulates appetite.[75] Ghrelin levels are diminished in *Helicobacter pylori* infection,[76] and it has been proposed that ghrelin may be the link between the decline in *H pylori* prevalence and the simultaneous increase in obesity and EAC seen in western populations in recent decades.[77] In this hypothesis, higher levels of ghrelin in subjects not infected with *H pylori* are proposed to cause appetite stimulation, weight gain, and increased risk of EAC; however, ghrelin concentrations are lower in obese than nonobese subjects,[78] and ghrelin also stimulates upper gastrointestinal motility,[79] which may decrease gastroesophageal reflux. It also has profound anti-inflammatory effects[80] and has been shown to cause a decrease in TNF-α–induced COX-2 and IL-1β expression in a BE cell line. It is biologically plausible that ghrelin may act to reduce EAC risk, and a prospective study undertaken within the Kaiser Permanente Health Plan supports a protective effect for high ghrelin levels against EAC. It is unlikely that ghrelin mediates the relationship between obesity and EAC risk.

SUMMARY

Evidence to date suggests that in whites and potentially Asians, obesity is associated with GERD symptoms, erosive reflux esophagitis, BE, and EAC in sporadic and familial cases. Obesity may impact the esophagitis-metaplasia-dysplasia-EAC sequence early by increasing the risk of erosive esophagitis. There is some evidence that the effect of obesity at this stage in the sequence may differ between whites and nonwhites and between the sexes. More work is necessary to understand why historically more obese populations have a lower risk of BE and EAC.

Recent evidence points to a more important role for abdominal versus overall obesity in the development of esophagitis. Overall obesity is associated with a modest increase in the risk of BE, but this may be mediated by abdominal obesity. There is no clear evidence that overall or abdominal obesity increases the risk of BE beyond that which results from an increase in its precursor, esophagitis. Weight loss in patients with GERD symptoms or esophagitis reduces reflux, improves their symptoms, and may improve the clinical and histologic presentation of esophagitis. Weight control and weight loss should be advised for patients with GERD symptoms and erosive esophagitis, even though there is no evidence that weight loss can prevent the development of BE in such patients.

Being overweight or obese is unquestionably a risk factor for EAC in whites, and abdominal adiposity appears to be at least as important a risk factor as general adiposity. At least part of the obesity-related EAC risk is mediated through an increase in gastroesophageal reflux and subsequent esophagitis, but a body of evidence is accruing that reflux-independent mechanisms are also important, such as the development of insulin resistance, alteration of the IGF pathway, and the production of leptin, adiponectin, and inflammatory cytokines by adipose tissue, especially visceral adipose tissue. Further exploration of the importance of abdominal or visceral adiposity in EAC risk is warranted, as is further examination of the role of adipokines in the development of this risk.

Two fundamental questions that are of relevance to the management of all BE patients remain unanswered: (1) whether being overweight or obese increases the risk of EAC and (2) whether weight loss can reduce this risk. Large prospective studies of BE patients with detailed anthropometric and radiologic measurements of fat distribution taken at baseline, with inclusion of appropriate surrogate measures of progression and with sufficient length of follow-up to enable EAC or high-grade dysplasia to be examined as outcomes, are required. Randomized trials of weight loss in BE patients will also be necessary, but such studies cannot, at present, be justified on the basis of current evidence.

REFERENCES

1. Blot WJ, McLaughlin JK. The changing epidemiology of esophageal cancer. Semin Orthod 1999;26(5 Suppl 15):2–8.
2. Conio M, Cameron AJ, Romero Y, et al. Secular trends in the epidemiology and outcome of Barrett's oesophagus in Olmsted County, Minnesota. Gut 2001; 48(3):304–9.
3. van Soest EM, Dieleman JP, Siersema PD, et al. Increasing incidence of Barrett's oesophagus in the general population. Gut 2005;54(8):1062–6.
4. Hampel H, Abraham NS, El-Serag HB. Meta-analysis: obesity and the risk for gastroesophageal reflux disease and its complications. Ann Intern Med 2005; 143(3):199–211.
5. Jacobson BC, Somers SC, Fuchs CS, et al. Body mass index and symptoms of gastroesophageal reflux in women. N Engl J Med 2006;354(22):2340–8.
6. Jung HK, Halder S, McNally M, et al. Overlap of gastro-oesophageal reflux disease and irritable bowel syndrome: prevalence and risk factors in the general population. Aliment Pharmacol Ther 2007;26(3):453–61.

7. Cremonini F, Locke GR III, Schleck CD, et al. Relationship between upper gastro-intestinal symptoms and changes in body weight in a population-based cohort. Neurogastroenterol Motil 2006;18(11):987–94.

8. Corley DA, Kubo A, Zhao W. Abdominal obesity, ethnicity and gastro-oesophageal reflux symptoms. Gut 2007;56(6):756–62.

9. Kang MS, Park DI, Oh SY, et al. Abdominal obesity is an independent risk factor for erosive esophagitis in a Korean population. J Gard Hist 2007;22(10):1656–61.

10. Lee HL, Eun CS, Lee OY, et al. Association between GERD-related erosive esophagitis and obesity. J Clin Gastroenterol 2008;42(6):672–5.

11. Kjellin A, Ramel S, Rossner S, et al. Gastroesophageal reflux in obese patients is not reduced by weight reduction. Scand J Gastroenterol 1996;31(11):1047–51.

12. Fraser-Moodie CA, Norton B, Gornall C, et al. Weight loss has an independent beneficial effect on symptoms of gastro-oesophageal reflux in patients who are overweight. Scand J Gastroenterol 1999;34(4):337–40.

13. Murray FE, Ennis J, Lennon JR, et al. Management of reflux oesophagitis: role of weight loss and cimetidine. Ir J Med Sci 1991;160(1):2–4.

14. Mathus-Vliegen EM, Tygat GN. Gastro-oesophageal reflux in obese subjects: influence of overweight, weight loss and chronic gastric balloon distension. Scand J Gastroenterol 2002;37(11):1246–52.

15. Reis GM, Savassi-Rocha PR, Nogueira AM, et al. Histological esophagitis before and after surgical treatment of morbid obesity (capella technique): a prospective study. Obes Surg 2008;18(4):367–70.

16. Stein DJ, El-Serag HB, Kuczynski J, et al. The association of body mass index with Barrett's oesophagus. Aliment Pharmacol Ther 2005;22(10):1005–10.

17. Bu X, Ma Y, Der R, et al. Body mass index is associated with Barrett esophagus and cardiac mucosal metaplasia. Dig Dis Sci 2006;51(9):1589–94.

18. Cook MB, Greenwood DC, Hardie LJ, et al. A systematic review and meta-analysis of the risk of increasing adiposity on Barrett's esophagus. Am J Gastroenterol 2008;103(2):292–300.

19. Anderson LA, Watson RG, Murphy SJ, et al. Risk factors for Barrett's oesophagus and oesophageal adenocarcinoma: results from the FINBAR study. World J Gastroenterol 2007;13(10):1585–94.

20. Smith KJ, O'Brien SM, Smithers BM, et al. Interactions among smoking, obesity, and symptoms of acid reflux in Barrett's esophagus. Cancer Epidemiol Biomarkers Prev 2005;14(11 Pt 1):2481–6.

21. Solaymani-Dodaran M, Logan RF, West J, et al. Risk of oesophageal cancer in Barrett's oesophagus and gastro-oesophageal reflux. Gut 2004;53(8):1070–4.

22. Edelstein ZR, Farrow DC, Bronner MP, et al. Central adiposity and risk of Barrett's esophagus. Gastroenterology 2007;133(2):403–11.

23. Corley DA, Kubo A, Levin TR, et al. Abdominal obesity and body mass index as risk factors for Barrett's esophagus. Gastroenterology 2007;133(1):34–41 [quiz 311].

24. Gerson LB, Ullah N, Fass R, et al. Does body mass index differ between patients with Barrett's oesophagus and patients with chronic gastro-oesophageal reflux disease? Aliment Pharmacol Ther 2007;25(9):1079–86.

25. Lagergren J, Bergstrom R, Nyren O. Association between body mass and adeno-carcinoma of the esophagus and gastric cardia. Ann Intern Med 1999;130(11):883–90.

26. Chow WH, Blot WJ, Vaughan TL, et al. Body mass index and risk of adenocarcinomas of the esophagus and gastric cardia. J Natl Cancer Inst 1998;90(2):150–5.

27. Corley DA, Kubo A, Zhao W. Abdominal obesity and the risk of esophageal and gastric cardia carcinomas. Cancer Epidemiol Biomarkers Prev 2008;17(2):352–8.

28. Kubo A, Corley DA. Body mass index and adenocarcinomas of the esophagus or gastric cardia: a systematic review and meta-analysis. Cancer Epidemiol Biomarkers Prev 2006;15(5):872–8.

29. Abnet CC, Freedman ND, Hollenbeck AR, et al. A prospective study of BMI and risk of oesophageal and gastric adenocarcinoma. Eur J Cancer 2008;44(3):465–71.

30. Renehan AG, Tyson M, Egger M, et al. Body mass index and incidence of cancer: a systematic review and meta-analysis of prospective observational studies. Lancet 2008;371(9612):569–78.

31. MacInnis RJ, English DR, Hopper JL, et al. Body size and composition and the risk of gastric and oesophageal adenocarcinoma. Int J Control 2006;118(10):2628–31.

32. Crane SJ, Locke GR III, Harmsen WS, et al. Subsite-specific risk factors for esophageal and gastric adenocarcinoma. Am J Gastroenterol 2007;102(8):1596–602.

33. Chak A, Lee T, Kinnard MF, et al. Familial aggregation of Barrett's oesophagus, oesophageal adenocarcinoma, and oesophagogastric junctional adenocarcinoma in Caucasian adults. Gut 2002;51(3):323–8.

34. Romero Y, Cameron AJ, Locke GR III, et al. Familial aggregation of gastroesophageal reflux in patients with Barrett's esophagus and esophageal adenocarcinoma. Gastroenterology 1997;113(5):1449–56.

35. de Jonge PJ, Steyerberg EW, Kuipers EJ, et al. Risk factors for the development of esophageal adenocarcinoma in Barrett's esophagus. Am J Gastroenterol 2006;101(7):1421–9.

36. Oberg S, Wenner J, Johansson J, et al. Barrett esophagus: risk factors for progression to dysplasia and adenocarcinoma. Ann Sci 2005;242(1):49–54.

37. Vaughan TL, Kristal AR, Blount PL, et al. Nonsteroidal anti-inflammatory drug use, body mass index, and anthropometry in relation to genetic and flow cytometric abnormalities in Barrett's esophagus. Cancer Epidemiol Biomarkers Prev 2002;11(8):745–52.

38. Risques RA, Vaughan TL, Li X, et al. Leukocyte telomere length predicts cancer risk in Barrett's esophagus. Cancer Epidemiol Biomarkers Prev 2007;16(12):2649–55.

39. Olliver JR, Hardie LJ, Gong Y, et al. Risk factors, DNA damage, and disease progression in Barrett's esophagus. Cancer Epidemiol Biomarkers Prev 2005;14(3):620–5.

40. Jin Z, Hamilton JP, Yang J, et al. Hypermethylation of the AKAP12 promoter is a biomarker of Barrett's-associated esophageal neoplastic progression. Cancer Epidemiol Biomarkers Prev 2008;17(1):111–7.

41. Jin Z, Olaru A, Yang J, et al. Hypermethylation of tachykinin-1 is a potential biomarker in human esophageal cancer. Clin Cancer Res 2007;13(21):6293–300.

42. Kristal AR, Blount PL, Schenk JM, et al. Low fat, high fruit and vegetable diets and weight loss do not affect biomarkers of cellular proliferation in Barrett esophagus. Cancer Epidemiol Biomarkers Prev 2005;14(10):2377–83.

43. Houghton SG, Romero Y, Sarr MG. Effect of Roux-en-Y gastric bypass in obese patients with Barrett's esophagus: attempts to eliminate duodenogastric reflux. Surg Obes Relat Dis 2008;4(1):1–4 [discussion: 4–5].

44. Stene-Larsen G, Weberg R, Froyshov Larsen I, et al. Relationship of overweight to hiatus hernia and reflux oesophagitis. Scand J Gastroenterol 1988;23(4):427–32.

45. Mercer CD, Wren SF, DaCosta LR, et al. Lower esophageal sphincter pressure and gastroesophageal pressure gradients in excessively obese patients. J Microencapsul 1987;18(3–4):135–46.

46. Mercer CD, Rue C, Hanelin L, et al. Effect of obesity on esophageal transit. Am J Sci 1985;149(1):177–81.

47. Wu JC, Mui LM, Cheung CM, et al. Obesity is associated with increased transient lower esophageal sphincter relaxation. Gastroenterology 2007;132(3):883–9.

48. El-Serag HB, Tran T, Richardson P, et al. Anthropometric correlates of intragastric pressure. Scand J Gastroenterol 2006;41(8):887–91.

49. Kershaw EE, Flier JS. Adipose tissue as an endocrine organ. J Clin Endocrinol Metab 2004;89(6):2548–56.

50. Vega GL, Adams-Huet B, Peshock R, et al. Influence of body fat content and distribution on variation in metabolic risk. J Clin Endocrinol Metab 2006;91(11):4459–66.

51. Renehan AG, Zwahlen M, Minder C, et al. Insulin-like growth factor (IGF)-I, IGF binding protein-3, and cancer risk: systematic review and meta-regression analysis. Lancet 2004;363(9418):1346–53.

52. Hankinson SE, Willett WC, Colditz GA, et al. Circulating concentrations of insulin-like growth factor-I and risk of breast cancer. Lancet 1998;351(9113):1393–6.

53. Chan JM, Stampfer MJ, Giovannucci E, et al. Plasma insulin-like growth factor-I and prostate cancer risk: a prospective study. Science 1998;279(5350):563–6.

54. Kaaks R, Toniolo P, Akhmedkhanov A, et al. Serum C-peptide, insulin-like growth factor (IGF)-I, IGF-binding proteins, and colorectal cancer risk in women. J Natl Cancer Inst 2000;92(19):1592–600.

55. Ma J, Pollak MN, Giovannucci E, et al. Prospective study of colorectal cancer risk in men and plasma levels of insulin-like growth factor (IGF)-I and IGF-binding protein-3. J Natl Cancer Inst 1999;91(7):620–5.

56. Cheng P, Gong J, Wang T, et al. Gene expression in rats with Barrett's esophagus and esophageal adenocarcinoma induced by gastroduodenoesophageal reflux. World J Gastroenterol 2005;11(33):5117–22.

57. Iravani S, Zhang HQ, Yuan ZQ, et al. Modification of insulin-like growth factor 1 receptor, c-Src, and Bcl-XL protein expression during the progression of Barrett's neoplasia. Hum Pathol 2003;34(10):975–82.

58. Di Martino E, Wild CP, Rotimi O, et al. IGFBP-3 and IGFBP-10 (CYR61) up-regulation during the development of Barrett's oesophagus and associated oesophageal adenocarcinoma: potential biomarkers of disease risk. Biomarkers 2006;11(6):547–61.

59. Siahpush SH, Vaughan TL, Lampe JN, et al. Longitudinal study of insulin-like growth factor, insulin-like growth factor binding protein-3, and their polymorphisms: risk of neoplastic progression in Barrett's esophagus. Cancer Epidemiol Biomarkers Prev 2007;16(11):2387–95.

60. Barb D, Williams CJ, Neuwirth AK, et al. Adiponectin in relation to malignancies: a review of existing basic research and clinical evidence. Am J Clin Nutr 2007;86(3):s858–66.

61. Tworoger SS, Eliassen AH, Kelesidis T, et al. Plasma adiponectin concentrations and risk of incident breast cancer. J Clin Endocrinol Metab 2007;92(4):1510–6.

62. Dal Maso L, Augustin LS, Karalis A, et al. Circulating adiponectin and endometrial cancer risk. J Clin Endocrinol Metab 2004;89(3):1160–3.

63. Cust AE, Kaaks R, Friedenreich C, et al. Plasma adiponectin levels and endometrial cancer risk in pre- and postmenopausal women. J Clin Endocrinol Metab 2007;92(1):255–63.

64. Wei EK, Giovannucci E, Fuchs CS, et al. Low plasma adiponectin levels and risk of colorectal cancer in men: a prospective study. J Natl Cancer Inst 2005;97(22): 1688–94.

65. Wolf AM, Wolf D, Rumpold H, et al. Adiponectin induces the anti-inflammatory cytokines IL-10 and IL-1RA in human leukocytes. Biochem Biophys Res Commun 2004;323(2):630–5.

66. Konturek PC, Burnat G, Rau T, et al. Effect of adiponectin and ghrelin on apoptosis of Barrett adenocarcinoma cell line. Dig Dis Sci 2008;53(3):597–605.

67. Kendall BJ, Macdonald GA, Hayward NK, et al. Leptin and the risk of Barrett's oesophagus. Gut 2008;57(4):448–54.

68. Thomas T, Burguera B, Melton LJ III, et al. Relationship of serum leptin levels with body composition and sex steroid and insulin levels in men and women. Metabolism 2000;49(10):1278–84.

69. Ogunwobi O, Mutungi G, Beales IL. Leptin stimulates proliferation and inhibits apoptosis in Barrett's esophageal adenocarcinoma cells by cyclooxygenase-2-dependent, prostaglandin-E2-mediated transactivation of the epidermal growth factor receptor and c-Jun NH2-terminal kinase activation. Endocrinology 2006; 147(9):4505–16.

70. Beales IL, Ogunwobi OO. Leptin synergistically enhances the anti-apoptotic and growth-promoting effects of acid in OE33 oesophageal adenocarcinoma cells in culture. Mol Cell Endocrinol 2007;274(1–2):60–8.

71. Francois F, Roper J, Goodman AJ, et al. The association of gastric leptin with oesophageal inflammation and metaplasia. Gut 2008;57(1):16–24.

72. Garofalo C, Surmacz E. Leptin and cancer. J Comp Psychol 2006;207(1):12–22.

73. Stattin P, Palmqvist R, Soderberg S, et al. Plasma leptin and colorectal cancer risk: a prospective study in northern Sweden. Oncol Rep 2003;10(6):2015–21.

74. Stattin P, Soderberg S, Biessy C, et al. Plasma leptin and breast cancer risk: a prospective study in northern Sweden. Breast Cancer Res Treat 2004;86(3): 191–6.

75. Wren AM, Seal LJ, Cohen MA, et al. Ghrelin enhances appetite and increases food intake in humans. J Clin Endocrinol Metab 2001;86(12):5992–5.

76. Isomoto H, Ueno H, Saenko VA, et al. Impact of *Helicobacter pylori* infection on gastric and plasma ghrelin dynamics in humans. Am J Gastroenterol 2005; 100(8):1711–20.

77. Nwokolo CU, Freshwater DA, O'Hare P, et al. Plasma ghrelin following cure of *Helicobacter pylori*. Gut 2003;52(5):637–40.

78. Tschop M, Weyer C, Tataranni PA, et al. Circulating ghrelin levels are decreased in human obesity. Diabetes 2001;50(4):707–9.

79. Dornonville de la Cour C, Lindstrom E, Norlen P, et al. Ghrelin stimulates gastric emptying but is without effect on acid secretion and gastric endocrine cells. Regul Pept 2004;120(1–3):23–32.

80. Dixit VD, Schaffer EM, Pyle RS, et al. Ghrelin inhibits leptin- and activation-induced proinflammatory cytokine expression by human monocytes and T cells. J Commun Inq 2004;114(1):57–66.

Molecular Markers and Genetics in Cancer Development

Kathy Hormi-Carver, PhD[a], Rhonda F. Souza, MD[a,b,*]

KEYWORDS

- Barrett's esophagus • Biomarkers
- Esophageal adenocarcinoma • Stem cell • Aneuploidy

One way in which organs in the gastrointestinal tract respond to chronic inflammation is through metaplasia, a process in which one adult cell type replaces another.[1,2] The metaplastic cells are thought to protect the tissue from the agents causing the inflammation. Metaplasia, however, may also predispose to malignancy. In the esophagus, chronic inflammation caused by gastroesophageal reflux disease results in replacement of the reflux-injured esophageal squamous cells by metaplastic, intestinal-type cells, a condition termed "Barrett's esophagus.[3,4]" Barrett's esophagus is the premalignant lesion for esophageal adenocarcinoma, a tumor whose incidence has risen at an alarming rate over the past three decades.[5]

In the traditional phenotypic model, carcinogenesis in Barrett's esophagus is envisioned as occurring in a step-wise progression from metaplasia to dysplasia and finally to adenocarcinoma. Endoscopic surveillance aimed at the detection of dysplasia remains the recommended strategy to detect early cancer progression in patients with Barrett's esophagus.[6] The use of dysplasia as an indicator of cancer progression is fraught with many problems, however, including poor intraobserver and interobserver reproducibility of dysplasia interpretations and poor predictive value in finding negative, indefinite, low-grade, and even high-grade dysplasia.[7–9] Dysplasia is essentially a constellation of histologic features suggesting that cells have acquired genetic abnormalities that render them neoplastic and predisposed to cancer formation.[1] Detection of the genetic abnormalities that allow a cell to manifest the morphologic features of dysplasia is an even earlier indicator of cancer progression. Recent interest has focused

[a] Division of Gastroenterology (111B1), Department of Medicine, VA North Texas Health Care System and the University of Texas Southwestern Medical School, 4500 South Lancaster Road, Dallas, TX 75216, USA
[b] Harold C. Simmons Comprehensive Cancer Center, University of Texas Southwestern Medical Center at Dallas, Dallas, TX, USA
* Corresponding author. Division of Gastroenterology (111B1), Department of Medicine, VA North Texas Health Care System and the University of Texas Southwestern Medical School, 4500 South Lancaster Road, Dallas, TX 75216.
E-mail address: rhonda.souza@utsouthwestern.edu (R.F. Souza).

Surg Oncol Clin N Am 18 (2009) 453–467
doi:10.1016/j.soc.2009.03.002
1055-3207/09/$ – see front matter. Published by Elsevier, Inc.

surgonc.theclinics.com

on the identification of molecular biomarkers, which may offer truly early detection of neoplastic progression and easy reproducibility and standardization.

The identification of biomarkers indicative of neoplasia developing in existing Barrett's esophagus requires an understanding of the molecular events that occur during the evolution of esophageal adenocarcinoma. In the genetic model of cancer progression, in contrast to the phenotypic model, cells progressively accumulate genetic abnormalities until they acquire six essential physiologic hallmarks of cancer originally proposed by Hanahan and Weinberg.[10] These physiologic cancer hallmarks include the ability to proliferate without exogenous stimulation; to resist growth-inhibitory signals; to avoid programmed cell death (apoptosis); to replicate without limit; to sustain new vascular supplies (angiogenesis); and to invade and metastasize.[10] To facilitate the acquisition of the numerous genetic abnormalities required to endow the cell with these essential hallmarks, tumor cells also display genomic instability, which increases the susceptibility of the genome to mutation.[10] This article focuses on the conceptual basis underlying the acquisition of each of the physiologic cancer hallmarks by metaplastic Barrett's cells (**Fig. 1**). The acquired genetic alterations that have shown the most promise as potential molecular biomarkers to predict neoplastic progression in patients with Barrett's esophagus are reviewed. Moreover, the role of stem cells and stem cell markers in Barrett's carcinogenesis is addressed.

PHYSIOLOGIC HALLMARKS OF CANCER
To Proliferate without Exogenous Stimulation

Normal cells require exogenous growth signals to undergo proliferation. In contrast, the ability of cancer cells to proliferate without exogenous stimulation was the first of the cancer hallmarks to be detailed by investigators.[10] In general, cellular proliferation requires passage through the phases of the cell cycle (**Fig. 2**). There are a number of checkpoints throughout the cell cycle, but the transition from G1 to S phase is perhaps the most well-studied and important. Early in G1, cell cycle progression is dependent on mitogenic signals. Once the cells enter S phase, mitogenic stimuli are no longer necessary and progression through the remainder of the cell cycle proceeds virtually automatically.[11]

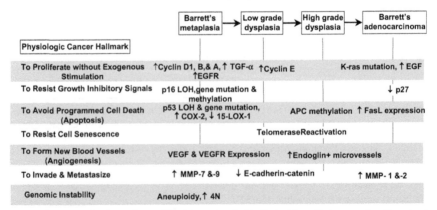

Fig. 1. Major genetic alterations allowing metaplastic Barrett's cells to acquire the physiologic hallmarks of cancer. Not all of the genetic alterations identified as Barrett's esophagus progresses to cancer are depicted. The approximate histologic stage at which each genetic change has been recognized is depicted.

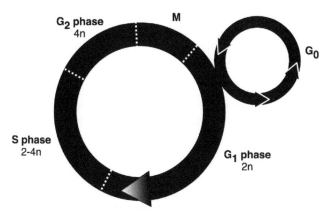

Fig. 2. The phases of the cell cycle. G0, quiescent state; G1, first gap; G2, second gap; M, mitosis; S, DNA synthesis; n, chromosome number.

Proto-oncogenes are normal cellular genes that promote growth. Oncogenes are simply these same proto-oncogenes that have become overactive because of mutation. Oncogenes can mimic many of the effects of normal growth signaling pathways, allowing the cells to proliferate without exogenous stimulation. In general, growth signals are normally transmitted into the cell by the binding of growth factors to growth factor receptors, which initiate intracellular signal transduction pathways resulting in the transmission of these growth-promoting signals to the nucleus. In the nucleus, these signals converge on pro-growth regulatory proteins that enhance cell proliferation by promoting progression from G1 to S phase of the cell cycle.

Alterations in growth factors, growth factor receptors, or the downstream signal transduction pathways activated in response to growth factor–receptor interactions have been found during the neoplastic progression of Barrett's cells. For example, increased expression of epidermal growth factor, transforming growth factor-α, and their receptor the epidermal growth factor receptor (also called ErbB-1) has been implicated in the development of Barrett's-associated adenocarcinomas.[12,13] The Ras/Raf/mitogen activated protein kinase pathway is one of the key growth factor–initiated intracellular signaling cascades.[14] Mutations in K-*ras* have been reported in 11% to 40% of esophageal adenocarcinomas, whereas oncogenic B-*raf* does not seem to play an important role.[15,16] Increased nuclear expression of pro-growth proteins that enhance progression from G1 to S phase of the cell cycle including cyclins D1, E, B1, and A has been found at various stages during the progression of metaplasia to esophageal adenocarcinoma.[17–20]

Potential molecular markers

Cyclins Cyclins A and D1 have been investigated as molecular biomarkers to predict neoplastic progression of Barrett's esophagus. In a small longitudinal case-control study, patients with surface expression of cyclin A in nondysplastic Barrett's biopsy tissues had a 7.6-fold higher risk of progression to either high-grade dysplasia or esophageal adenocarcinoma than biopsy tissues from those patients where surface expression of cyclin A was not detected.[20] Likewise, staining for cyclin D1 has been found in 67% of biopsies of nondysplastic Barrett's mucosa in those patients who progressed to esophageal adenocarcinoma compared with expression in only 29% of biopsies from those Barrett's patients who did not develop esophageal adenocarcinoma (odds ratio, 6.85).[21] In a subsequent larger, population-based case-control study, however, cyclin D1 expression did not seem to predict neoplastic progression in patients with Barrett's esophagus.[22] Although these results are promising, the discordant findings regarding the use of cyclin D1 as a potential biomarker highlight the need for large-scale prospective clinical trials before recommending widespread clinical use of the cyclins as biomarkers.

To Resist Growth-Inhibitory Signals

Similar to the growth stimulatory signals, growth inhibitory signals are transmitted by surface receptors to intracellular signal transduction cascades, which in turn transmit these signals to the nucleus. Integration of these growth inhibitory signals in the nucleus blocks cell proliferation by preventing passage from G1 into S phase of the cell cycle. In general, it is the function of tumor suppressor genes to block cell proliferation. If tumor cells are to burgeon then they must inactivate tumor suppressor genes and avoid these growth inhibitory signals. There are at least three mechanisms whereby tumor cells can inactivate tumor suppressor genes: (1) mutation; (2) deletion of the chromosomal region containing the gene (loss of heterozygosity [LOH]); or (3) attachment of methyl groups to the promoter region of genes (promoter hypermethylation). During neoplastic progression, Barrett's cells have demonstrated inactivation of tumor suppressor genes by each of these mechanisms.

Examples of tumor suppressor genes inactivated during the neoplastic progression of Barrett's esophagus include p53, p16, p27, and the adenomatous polyposis coli (APC) gene. Normally, p16 and p53 act to prevent cell growth by blocking progression from G1 to S phase of the cell cycle. If these genes are inactivated, dysregulated cell proliferation can occur. Numerous studies demonstrate frequent inactivation of p16 and p53 during the neoplastic progression of Barrett's esophagus. For example, loss of 9p21, the chromosomal locus for p16, has been found in approximately 82% of esophageal adenocarcinomas, whereas methylation of the p16 promoter occurs in 45% of cases.[23] Moreover, genetic alterations of p16 are among the earliest events in the neoplastic progression of Barrett's esophagus with promoter methylation, LOH, or mutation found in 73% to 87% of metaplastic Barrett's biopsies.[24,25] p53 is also frequently inactivated by loss of 17p, the p53 locus, and mutation of p53 on the remaining allele in approximately 50% to 90% of esophageal adenocarcinomas.[26–28] Unlike the classic molecular "adenoma-carcinoma" sequence of genetic alterations in colorectal carcinoma, the key molecular events at each stage of neoplastic progression in Barrett's esophagus are not well delineated. Genetic ordering becomes important when trying to identify molecular biomarkers early in the process of neoplastic progression to which diagnostic tests or therapeutic interventions can be directed. Although clinical data are limited on the order of genetic alterations underlying carcinogenesis in Barrett's esophagus, Maley and colleagues[25] reported that only 3% of biopsies of nondysplastic Barrett's esophagus contained alterations in p53 that did not also contain alterations in p16, suggesting that p16 is one of the earliest genes targeted for inactivation in Barrett's esophagus.

Other tumor suppressor proteins, such as p27 and APC, block cell proliferation by inhibiting proteins that are involved in cellular signaling. For example, p27 normally prevents passage from G1 to S phase by inhibiting cyclin E. Loss of p27 protein expression has been found in 83% of esophageal adenocarcinomas, and has been correlated with aggressive tumor behavior and poor patient outcomes.[29] APC normally inhibits cell proliferation by binding with and targeting the pro-proliferative transcription factor β-catenin for degradation. Inactivation of APC prevents the destruction of β-catenin thereby allowing this protein to enter the nucleus and mediate the expression of several growth-related genes whose protein products promote passage from G1 into S phase of the cell cycle.[30,31] Although mutation of APC has only rarely been reported, LOH of 5q21, the APC locus, has been found in approximately 45% of esophageal adenocarcinomas.[32] A more common mechanism for altering APC expression is promoter hypermethylation, which has been reported in more than 80% of Barrett's high-grade dysplasias and esophageal adenocarcinomas and 40% to 50% of nondysplastic Barrett's metaplasias.[33–35]

Potential molecular markers

17p Loss of heterozygosity and p53 mutation LOH of 17p, the locus for p53, has been investigated as a potential marker to predict cancer progression in Barrett's esophagus. In a large, longitudinal, prospective study, 17p LOH was a significant predictor of cancer progression at 5 years in Barrett's patients whose grade of dysplasia ranged from no dysplasia to high-grade dysplasia.[36] Furthermore, the ability of 17p LOH to predict progression to high-grade dysplasia or cancer remained significant when only those Barrett's patients whose biopsies demonstrated no dysplasia, indefinite dysplasia, or low-grade dysplasia were assessed.[36] Recent data from this same group have confirmed the ability of 17p LOH to predict neoplastic progression of Barrett's esophagus.[37] Although not as strong a predictor as 17p LOH, p53 mutation was also found to predict progression to cancer.[37] Well-designed, prospective, clinical studies are still needed, however, to estimate the reduction in cancer formation of identifying 17p LOH in biopsies of Barrett's epithelium before this potential biomarker is put into widespread clinical use.

In addition to using a molecular biomarker that accurately predicts cancer progression, the assay used to detect the biomarker must be reliable, feasible, and validated. For example, in the studies discussed previously, 17p LOH was detected by flow cytometric analysis, a technique that is not widely available. If a technique that is more practical for widespread clinical use were available, however, then movement of 17p LOH into the clinics might become more feasible. Fluorescence in situ hybridization (FISH) is a routine technique that can be used to detect LOH. FISH has been used on biopsy tissues and on brush cytology specimens of Barrett's esophagus in a number of cross-sectional studies to detect 17p LOH during the neoplastic progression of Barrett's esophagus with promising results.[38–41] In a study by Rygiel and colleagues,[41] FISH detected loss of 17p in brush cytology samples from 5% of patients with nondysplastic Barrett's mucosa, 9% of those with low-grade dysplasia, and 46% of those with high-grade dysplasia suggesting that FISH may be an alternative to flow cytometry to detect LOH. A head-to-head comparison of FISH and flow cytometry, however, demonstrated a lower sensitivity for FISH in detecting 17p LOH when applied to esophagectomy tissue samples from Barrett's patients undergoing surgery for high-grade dysplasia or esophageal adenocarcinoma.[39] Because FISH and flow cytometry are not equivalent in their ability to detect 17p LOH, larger longitudinal studies using FISH in patients with Barrett's esophagus are needed before considering it as a clinically useful biomarker assay.[39]

9p Loss of heterozygosity, methylated p16, and p16 mutation In a large prospective study, alterations in p16 by LOH, promoter methylation, and mutation have been investigated as individual biomarkers in Barrett's esophagus. Galipeau and colleagues[37] found that the 10-year incidence of cancer was 19% in patients whose biopsies of Barrett's mucosa demonstrated 9p LOH compared with 7% in those patients whose biopsies did not. In contrast, the finding of methylation of p16 or p16 mutation in biopsies of Barrett's mucosa was not a significant predicator of cancer progression.[37] As discussed later, it seems that 9p LOH may be most useful when used in combination with other molecular biomarkers rather than being used alone as a single marker in patients with Barrett's esophagus.

p53 Antibodies and methylated the adenomatous polyposis coli DNA in plasma In patients with Barrett's esophagus who progressed to cancer, p53 antibodies could be detected in the serum before the cancer diagnosis suggesting that serologic biomarkers, like tissue biomarkers, may be useful to identify a subset of patients at risk for neoplastic progression.[42] Although methylated APC DNA has not been investigated as a predictive biomarker in patients with Barrett's esophagus, detecting it in the plasma of patients with esophageal adenocarcinoma has been associated with a significantly shortened survival.[34] These results are promising, but large-scale prospective studies are still needed to validate the use of serologic biomarkers as predictive or prognostic indicators in patients with Barrett's esophagus and esophageal adenocarcinoma.

To Avoid Programmed Cell Death (Apoptosis)

Tumor cell expansion is regulated not only by the rate of cell proliferation, but also by the rate of cell death. The apoptotic program is present in all normal cells and once the program is initiated, it proceeds in a series of well-choreographed events culminating in cell destruction. To normal cells, apoptosis is a protective mechanism because it prevents cells with damaged DNA from undergoing replication. To cancer cells, however, apoptosis is a barrier that must be overcome. The apoptotic program can be initiated by the activation of death receptors; a disruption in the cell's well-being (ie, DNA damage, oncogene activation, metabolic abnormalities); or by the loss of cell-cell or cell-matrix contact.[10] Regardless of how the program is initiated, the caspases, a family of intracellular proteases, are the ultimate effectors of cell death.[43]

Barrett's-associated adenocarcinomas have found a variety of ways to avoid apoptosis. For example, inactivation of p53 is one way in which Barrett's cancer cells can avoid inducing apoptosis triggered by DNA damage, metabolic abnormalities, or oncogene activation. Barrett's cancer cells have also been found to alter the expression levels of enzymes whose products influence the rate of apoptosis. Expression of 15-lipoxygenase-1, whose product 13-S-hydroxyoctadecadienoic acid triggers apoptosis, has been found to decrease and the expression of cycloxygenase-2 (COX-2), whose prostaglandin products inhibit apoptosis, has been found to increase in esophageal adenocarcinomas.[44–46] Finally, Barrett's cancer cells can also avoid activating death receptors, such as Fas.[47] The binding of Fas-ligand, a death-promoting ligand, to its cell surface receptor Fas initiates the apoptotic program.[47] Normally, FasL is expressed by activated lymphocytes, whereas the Fas receptor is on both lymphocytes and epithelial cells. By expressing FasL, tumor cells now acquire the ability to initiate apoptosis in the Fas receptor expressing lymphocytes, avoiding immune destruction. In one study of 13 esophageal adenocarcinomas, all were found to express FasL as detected by immunohistochemical staining.[48]

Potential molecular markers

COX-2 expression There has been a lot of attention focused on selective inhibition of COX-2 as a chemopreventive strategy in Barrett's esophagus; however, COX-2 has also been investigated as a possible biomarker to predict neoplastic progression. A case control study from the United Kingdom found no association between COX-2 staining in biopsies of Barrett's metaplasia and progression to either high-grade dysplasia or esophageal adenocarcinoma.[22] Positive staining for COX-2 and p53 in the metaplastic Barrett's biopsies was associated with a markedly increased risk for neoplastic progression (odds ratio, 27.3); however, staining for this combination of proteins was found in only 15% of the patients who progressed to dysplasia or adenocarcinoma.[22] In a population-based case control study, Ferguson and colleagues[49] evaluated whether the COX-2 8473 T>C polymorphism, located in the promoter region of the COX-2 gene, was associated with reflux esophagitis, Barrett's esophagus, or esophageal adenocarcinoma. The presence of one COX-2 8473 C allele was associated with an increased risk of esophageal adenocarcinoma (adjusted odds ratio, 1.58), but not with reflux esophagitis or Barrett's esophagus.[49]

To Resist Cell Senescence

Acquisition of the three hallmarks discussed previously allows cells to proliferate independent of extrinsic environmental signals. Normal cells, however, also contain intrinsic mechanisms that limit their proliferative capacity. To become immortal, the cells must overcome this autonomous, intrinsic mechanism for cell senescence, a process that involves the loss of telomeres. Telomeres are long stretches of a repetitive DNA sequences located on the ends of chromosomes. Each time the cell divides, some of these telomeric DNA repeats are lost. Eventually, when the telomeres become too short, the cells exit from the cell cycle at G1 and enter G0, a permanent growth arrest termed "senescence." Cells must maintain their telomere length to become immortal. Telomerase is the enzyme that allows cells to maintain their telomeres.[50] Unlike most normal somatic cells, tumor cells often express telomerase. Most normal esophageal squamous cells lack telomerase, whereas metaplastic Barrett's cells express low levels of telomerase, which increases as the cells progress to high-grade dysplasia.[51] High levels of telomerase expression have also been found in esophageal adenocarcinomas.[52]

Potential molecular markers

Telomerase Telomerase expression has a number of features desirable in a molecular biomarker. Telomerase is undetectable in most normal esophageal squamous cells. Moreover, data suggest that telomerase expression increases in a step-wise fashion as metaplastic Barrett's cells develop increasingly severe grades of dysplasia, with very high levels found in Barrett's-associated adenocarcinomas. In a cross-sectional study, telomerase activity was found to be significantly higher in esophageal adenocarcinomas compared with metaplastic Barrett's esophagus. Human telomerase reverse-transcriptase (hTERT) mRNA levels were not significantly different, however, suggesting that alterations in hTERT gene transcription were not responsible for the observed difference in telomerase activity.[53] In a small, longitudinal, prospective study, hypermethylation of the hTERT promoter was found in 92% of samples of Barrett's mucosa from patients who progressed to esophageal adenocarcinoma compared with 17% in samples from those Barrett's patients who did not develop cancer, suggesting that hTERT promoter hypermethylation may be a potential marker to identify those patients who are at risk for cancer progression.[54] Promoter hypermethylation is one way in which gene transcription can be reduced. The data from Barclay and colleagues[53] suggest that hTERT mRNA levels do not correlate with telomerase activity and that it is telomerase activity that increases during neoplastic progression of Barrett's esophagus, findings that may limit the use of hTERT promoter methylation as a meaningful predictive biomarker. Large-scale prospective studies are needed to validate the use of telomerase activity and hTERT promoter hypermethylation as predictive biomarkers for cancer risk in patients with Barrett's esophagus.

To Sustain New Vascular Supplies (Angiogenesis)

The formation of new blood vessels (angiogenesis) is essential to provide nutrients and oxygen and eliminate metabolic waste products from growing tumors. The vascular endothelial growth factors (VEGFs) and their receptors, the vascular endothelial growth factor receptors (VEGFRs), initiate the angiogenic signals. Once triggered, these angiogenic signals result in the proliferation and migration of endothelial cells into the tumor.

The epithelial cells of metaplastic Barrett's esophagus have been found to express VEGF-A, VEGF-C, and VEGFR-2, the corresponding receptor for VEGF-A, whereas neoplastic Barrett's tissues demonstrate VEGFR-3.[55,56] It has been proposed that the salmon color characteristic of Barrett's esophagus results from its enriched vascular network. Esophageal adenocarcinomas express significantly higher levels of VEGF mRNA and protein expression compared with normal esophageal mucosa, metaplastic and dysplastic Barrett's esophagus, and normal esophageal mucosa.[57] Endothelial cells involved in tumor angiogenesis express the receptor endoglin.[58] Barrett's epithelium with high-grade dysplasia has been found with a significantly greater number of endoglin-staining microvessels than Barrett's with low-grade dysplasia.[58] Moreover, in those patients with esophageal adenocarcinoma, the number of tumor microvessels that stain with endoglin has been found to correlate significantly with angiolymphatic invasion, lymph node metastasis, and overall prognosis.[58] Although VEGF and endoglin expression may serve as prognostic markers for patients with high-grade dysplasia in Barrett's esophagus and esophageal adenocarcinoma, no data exist for a role of these markers to predict the risk of cancer progression in patients with metaplastic Barrett's esophagus.

To Invade and Metastasize

The ability to invade and metastasize are complex processes whose mechanisms remain incompletely understood; however, disruptions in proteins involved in anchoring cells within a tissue and in extracellular proteases are thought to play a role.[10] Alterations in cell-cell adhesion molecules, such as E-cadherin and β-catenin, and in integrins, which attach cells to the extracellular matrix, are frequently involved in disrupting the anchoring of cells. Normally, E-cadherin and β-catenin are located at the cell surface membrane allowing cells to adhere to each other, allowing the transmission of antigrowth signals. When these proteins are disrupted, cells are predisposed to invasion and metastasis. Decreased membranous staining for E-cadherin and β-catenin and increased cytoplasmic and nuclear staining of these proteins, respectively, have been found as the degree of dysplasia increases in Barrett's epithelium.[59,60] Matrix metalloproteinases (MMPs) are proteolytic enzymes capable of destroying the extracellular matrix, facilitating tumor invasion and metastasis.[61] Expression of MMP-1, -2, -7, and -9 has been associated with Barrett's esophagus and esophageal adenocarcinoma.[62–64] Matrilysin (MMP-7) has been found to be the primary MMP in Barrett's esophagus and esophageal adenocarcinoma and its expression was correlated with tumor aggressiveness as determined by histologic criteria.[64]

Potential molecular markers

β-catenin and E-cadherin   Only a few studies have investigated the use of β-catenin and E-cadherin as predictive or prognostic markers in Barrett's esophagus and esophageal adenocarcinoma. In a case control study, Murray and colleagues[22] found no association between β-catenin staining in biopsies of Barrett's metaplasia and progression to either high-grade dysplasia or esophageal adenocarcinoma. In a study of 59 cases of Barrett's-associated esophageal adenocarcinoma, absent membranous staining for E-cadherin, but not β-catenin, predicted a worse outcome.[65] One potential explanation for the absence of membrane staining of β-catenin to demonstrate use as a prognostic indicator may be that this abnormal staining pattern was found in early stage esophageal adenocarcinomas (Tis–T1), whereas the later stage tumors (T2–T3) demonstrate intact, membranous β-catenin expression.[66]

Matrix metalloproteinases No studies have yet investigated whether MMP expression may predict neoplastic progression in patients with Barrett's esophagus. The expression of MMPs in esophageal tumors has been found, however, to correlate with lymphatic invasion, lymph node metastasis, and overall prognosis.[63]

Genomic Instability Facilitates Acquisition of the Cancer Hallmarks

Changes in the genomes of cells are needed for them to acquire the physiologic hallmarks of cancer cells. The inactivation of individual genes is an inefficient process, however, particularly because the cell contains a complex array of DNA damage warning and repair systems, which function to maintain genomic integrity.[10] The genomes of cancer cells must become unstable for tumors to occur. Genomic instability can manifest as abnormalities in chromosomal content that occur because of losses or gains in whole chromosomes or in segments of chromosomes. Aneuploidy indicates a cell whose chromosomal content is abnormal in that it is other than the normal diploid (2n) or tetraploid (4n) (where n equals chromosomal number). The finding of aneuploidy suggests that the risk of neoplastic progression may be increased. Moreover, aneuploidy reflects widespread cellular DNA damage rather than a single gene mutation.

Potential molecular markers

Aneuploidy Aneuploidy can be detected clinically by flow cytometry and by FISH. In a large prospective study, the detection of aneuploidy or the fraction of tetraploid cell populations (4N) by flow cytometry predicted neoplastic progression of Barrett's esophagus.[67] Although tetraploid cell populations within tissues are normal, if more than 6% of the total cell population demonstrates tetraploidy than the tissue is at an increased risk for cancer progression.[67,68] The 5-year incidence of cancer was 64% in patients with aneuploidy (populations with over 2.7N) detected in their biopsies of Barrett's mucosa; 57% in patients with 4n fractions (tetraploidy) over 6%; and 75% in patients with both aneuploidy and tetraploidy.[9,67] In patients whose biopsies did not demonstrate aneuploidy or tetraploidy, the risk of developing cancer was only 5.2% and all of these patients had high-grade dysplasia in their biopsies.[67] The finding of aneuploidy or tetraploidy in biopsies demonstrating high-grade dysplasia, however, did not add to the already high predictive value of the histologic diagnosis of high-grade dysplasia itself. Rather, the detection of aneuploidy and tetraploidy was most helpful in predicting cancer progression in patients whose biopsies demonstrated no dysplasia, indefinite dysplasia, or low-grade dysplasia. In these patients, the 5-year incidence of cancer was 39% if their biopsies demonstrated either aneuploidy or tetraploidy compared with 0% in patients whose biopsies did not contain either of these flow cytometric abnormalities.[67] The finding that aneuploidy can predict neoplastic progression in patients with Barrett's esophagus has been confirmed by other investigators in a recent study.[69]

In addition to flow cytometry, FISH can also be used to detect aneuploidy; however, the caveats noted previously for this technique still remain.[70] Image cytometry has been proposed to be more sensitive than flow cytometry in detecting aneuploidy.[71,72] Recently, this technique has become automated and it seems to be more sensitive than standard flow cytometry in detecting aneuploidy in Barrett's-associated esophageal adenocarcinomas.[73] The detection of aneuploidy by any of these techniques has not been tested in large, prospective clinical trials, however, to determine if this biomarker actually reduces the risk of cancer formation in patients with Barrett's esophagus.

The combination of aneuploidy-tetraploidy, 17p loss of heterozygosity, and 9p loss of heterozygosity In a large prospective study, the ability of these individual biomarkers alone or in combination to detect cancer progression in patients with Barrett's esophagus was determined. At 10 years, the incidence of cancer was approximately 20% in those patients whose biopsies demonstrated one of these abnormalities and 36% in those whose biopsies demonstrated two abnormalities.[37] For patients whose biopsies contained all three abnormalities, the cancer incidence was 80% at 6 years.[37] In those patients whose biopsies did not show any of these abnormalities, the incidence of cancer was 12% at the end of 10 years.[37] A panel of biomarkers rather than any one individual biomarker may be better at predicting neoplastic progression of Barrett's esophagus and large, prospective clinical trials are eagerly awaited.

STEM CELLS, STEM CELL MARKERS, AND CARCINOGENESIS IN BARRETT'S ESOPHAGUS

Esophageal adenocarcinoma arises in Barrett's esophagus at a rate of approximately 0.5% per year.[74] Persistence of the metaplastic epithelial lining of the esophagus places individuals at continued risk for cancer formation. Maintenance of this metaplastic epithelium requires continued epithelial cell renewal by stem cells, which have the unique property of self-renewal. Self-renewal is the process whereby when the stem cell divides it gives rise not only to a progenitor cell but also to another stem cell. It is the progenitor cell that undergoes rapid proliferation and differentiation as it migrates toward the luminal surface. The stem cell that gives rise to the stratified squamous epithelium has been potentially identified by the putative stem cell marker p63.[75] The stem cell that gives rise to Barrett's metaplasia has not yet been identified, however, likely because of the lack of reliable stem cell markers. Recently, leucine-rich-repeat-containing G-protein-coupled receptor 5 (Lgr5), whose gene is a downstream target of the Wnt signaling pathway, and doublecortin and CaM kinase-like-1 (DCAMKL-1), a microtubule-associated kinase, have been proposed as putative markers for intestinal stem cells.[76,77] Because Barrett's metaplasia is a form of incomplete intestinal metaplasia, perhaps these putative intestinal stem cell markers might also identify the stem cells in Barrett's esophagus.

For years, cancers of the gastrointestinal tract have been thought to arise through clonal evolution, the process in which cells acquire genetic alterations in a stepwise fashion that endow them with a growth advantage over neighboring cells.[78] Depending on the number and types of genetic alterations, various clones of cells exist within the tumor, each having a different propensity for survival compared with neighboring clones and each maintaining some capacity for self-renewal.[78] Recently, the concept of cancer stem cells has gained increased attention. In contrast to the model of clonal evolution, the stem cell model proposes that tumor growth, like normal tissue growth, is sustained by only a few stem cells and that most cells within the tumor have no capacity for self-renewal.[78]

The current approach to identifying molecular markers indicative of neoplastic progression in Barrett's esophagus is based on the clonal evolution concept of tumor formation. If the cancer stem cell concept is correct, however, then perhaps it is the metaplastic Barrett's stem cell that sustains the initial pro-proliferative genetic alterations. This growth-advantaged cell is now capable of self-renewal and gives rise to progenitor cells, which can sustain additional genetic alterations and manifest abhorrent patterns of differentiation that perhaps result in the phenotypic changes recognized pathologically as dysplasia. Additional mutations in these "dysplastic" stem cells may give rise to "cancer" stem cells that initiate and sustain the resulting esophageal adenocarcinoma.[79] Preventing and eliminating cancer in Barrett's esophagus could be achieved by destroying the Barrett's stem cell.[80] If markers, such as Lgr5 and DCAMKL-1, can identify those stem cells, then it might be possible to target endoscopic ablative or pharmacologic therapies specifically to the stem cells, doing away with Barrett's esophagus and esophageal adenocarcinoma.

SUMMARY

The incidence of esophageal adenocarcinoma has risen at an alarming rate over the past several decades. Barrett's esophagus is one of the major risk factors for esophageal adenocarcinoma and using molecular markers to identify the subset of Barrett's patients at risk for cancer progression has been a subject of intense interest. It has become increasingly important to understand the pathogenesis of esophageal adenocarcinoma and Barrett's esophagus at the molecular level to identify potential biomarkers. Although only a fraction of the genetic alterations required for benign, metaplastic Barrett's cells to acquire the physiologic hallmarks of cancer are reviewed in this article, it is hoped that the conceptual basis for selecting potential molecular biomarkers has been established. Although the routine clinical use of biomarkers is not yet recommended, it seems reasonable to assume that biomarker validation studies will be performed in the coming years and that movement into the clinics is inevitable. Also, continuing progress in identifying intestinal stem cell markers will likely allow for the identification of Barrett's stem cells. Ablation of these stem cells by pharmacologic or endoscopic therapies may prevent the development of Barrett's esophagus and halt the rising incidence of esophageal adenocarcinoma.

ACKNOWLEDGMENTS

We are grateful to Dr. Stuart J. Spechler for his thoughtful review of the manuscript and helpful suggestions and to Mr. Jim Hardy for his assistance with the illustrations.

REFERENCES

1. Spechler SJ. Intestinal metaplasia at the gastroesophageal junction. Gastroenterology 2004;126:567–75.
2. Tosh D, Slack JM. How cells change their phenotype. Nat Rev Mol Cell Biol 2002; 3:187–94.
3. Spechler SJ. Clinical practice. Barrett's esophagus. N Engl J Med 2002;346: 836–42.
4. Lagergren J, Bergstrom R, Lindgren A, et al. Symptomatic gastroesophageal reflux as a risk factor for esophageal adenocarcinoma. N Engl J Med 1999;340: 825–31.
5. Pohl H, Welch HG. The role of overdiagnosis and reclassification in the marked increase of esophageal adenocarcinoma incidence. J Natl Cancer Inst 2005; 97:142–6.
6. Wang KK, Sampliner RE. Updated guidelines 2008 for the diagnosis, surveillance and therapy of Barrett's esophagus. Am J Gastroenterol 2008;103:788–97.
7. Reid BJ, Haggitt RC, Rubin CE, et al. Observer variation in the diagnosis of dysplasia in Barrett's esophagus. Hum Pathol 1988;19:166–78.
8. Montgomery E, Bronner MP, Goldblum JR, et al. Reproducibility of the diagnosis of dysplasia in Barrett esophagus: a reaffirmation. Hum Pathol 2001;32:368–78.

9. Reid BJ, Levine DS, Longton G, et al. Predictors of progression to cancer in Barrett's esophagus: baseline histology and flow cytometry identify low- and high-risk patient subsets. Am J Gastroenterol 2000;95:1669–76.

10. Hanahan D, Weinberg RA. The hallmarks of cancer. Cell 2000;100:57–70.

11. Lundberg AS, Weinberg RA. Control of the cell cycle and apoptosis. Eur J Cancer 1999;35:531–9.

12. Jankowski J, Hopwood D, Wormsley KG. Flow-cytometric analysis of growth-regulatory peptides and their receptors in Barrett's oesophagus and oesophageal adenocarcinoma. Scand J Gastroenterol 1992;27:147–54.

13. Brito MJ, Filipe MI, Linehan J, et al. Association of transforming growth factor alpha (TGFA) and its precursors with malignant change in Barrett's epithelium: biological and clinical variables. Int J Cancer 1995;60:27–32.

14. Malumbres M, Pellicer A. RAS pathways to cell cycle control and cell transformation. Front Biosci 1998;3:d887–912.

15. Lord RV, O'Grady R, Sheehan C, et al. K-ras codon 12 mutations in Barrett's oesophagus and adenocarcinomas of the oesophagus and oesophagogastric junction. J Gastroenterol Hepatol 2000;15:730–6.

16. Sommerer F, Vieth M, Markwarth A, et al. Mutations of BRAF and KRAS2 in the development of Barrett's adenocarcinoma. Oncogene 2004;23:554–8.

17. Arber N, Lightdale C, Rotterdam H, et al. Increased expression of the cyclin D1 gene in Barrett's esophagus. Cancer Epidemiol Biomarkers Prev 1996;5:457–9.

18. Sarbia M, Bektas N, Muller W, et al. Expression of cyclin E in dysplasia, carcinoma, and nonmalignant lesions of Barrett esophagus. Cancer 1999;86:2597–601.

19. Geddert H, Heep HJ, Gabbert HE, et al. Expression of cyclin B1 in the metaplasia-dysplasia-carcinoma sequence of Barrett esophagus. Cancer 2002;94:212–8.

20. Lao-Sirieix P, Lovat L, Fitzgerald RC. Cyclin A immunocytology as a risk stratification tool for Barrett's esophagus surveillance. Clin Cancer Res 2007;13:659–65.

21. Bani-Hani K, Martin IG, Hardie LJ, et al. Prospective study of cyclin D1 overexpression in Barrett's esophagus: association with increased risk of adenocarcinoma. J Natl Cancer Inst 2000;92:1316–21.

22. Murray L, Sedo A, Scott M, et al. TP53 and progression from Barrett's metaplasia to oesophageal adenocarcinoma in a UK population cohort. Gut 2006;55:1390–7.

23. Wong DJ, Barrett MT, Stoger R, et al. p16INK4a promoter is hypermethylated at a high frequency in esophageal adenocarcinomas. Cancer Res 1997;57:2619–22.

24. Wong DJ, Paulson TG, Prevo LJ, et al. p16(INK4a) lesions are common, early abnormalities that undergo clonal expansion in Barrett's metaplastic epithelium. Cancer Res 2001;61:8284–9.

25. Maley CC, Galipeau PC, Li X, et al. The combination of genetic instability and clonal expansion predicts progression to esophageal adenocarcinoma. Cancer Res 2004;64:7629–33.

26. Hamelin R, Flejou JF, Muzeau F, et al. TP53 gene mutations and p53 protein immunoreactivity in malignant and premalignant Barrett's esophagus. Gastroenterology 1994;107:1012–8.

27. Galipeau PC, Prevo LJ, Sanchez CA, et al. Clonal expansion and loss of heterozygosity at chromosomes 9p and 17p in premalignant esophageal (Barrett's) tissue. J Natl Cancer Inst 1999;91:2087–95.

28. Meltzer SJ, Yin J, Huang Y, et al. Reduction to homozygosity involving p53 in esophageal cancers demonstrated by the polymerase chain reaction. Proc Natl Acad Sci U S A 1991;88:4976–80.

29. Singh SP, Lipman J, Goldman H, et al. Loss or altered subcellular localization of p27 in Barrett's associated adenocarcinoma. Cancer Res 1998;58:1730–5.
30. Huber O, Korn R, McLaughlin J, et al. Nuclear localization of beta-catenin by interaction with transcription factor LEF-1. Mech Dev 1996;59:3–10.
31. Rubinfeld B, Albert I, Porfiri E, et al. Binding of GSK3beta to the APC-beta-catenin complex and regulation of complex assembly. Science 1996;272:1023–6.
32. Dolan K, Garde J, Walker SJ, et al. LOH at the sites of the DCC, APC, and TP53 tumor suppressor genes occurs in Barrett's metaplasia and dysplasia adjacent to adenocarcinoma of the esophagus. Hum Pathol 1999;30:1508–14.
33. Eads CA, Lord RV, Kurumboor SK, et al. Fields of aberrant CpG island hypermethylation in Barrett's esophagus and associated adenocarcinoma. Cancer Res 2000;60:5021–6.
34. Kawakami K, Brabender J, Lord RV, et al. Hypermethylated APC DNA in plasma and prognosis of patients with esophageal adenocarcinoma. J Natl Cancer Inst 2000;92:1805–11.
35. Clement G, Jablons DM, Benhattar J. Targeting the Wnt signaling pathway to treat Barrett's esophagus. Expert Opin Ther Targets 2007;11:375–89.
36. Reid BJ, Prevo LJ, Galipeau PC, et al. Predictors of progression in Barrett's esophagus II: baseline 17p (p53) loss of heterozygosity identifies a patient subset at increased risk for neoplastic progression. Am J Gastroenterol 2001; 96:2839–48.
37. Galipeau PC, Li X, Blount PL, et al. NSAIDs modulate CDKN2A, TP53, and DNA content risk for progression to esophageal adenocarcinoma. PLoS Med 2007;4: 342–54.
38. Fahmy M, Skacel M, Gramlich TL, et al. Chromosomal gains and genomic loss of p53 and p16 genes in Barrett's esophagus detected by fluorescence in situ hybridization of cytology specimens. Mod Pathol 2004;17:588–96.
39. Wongsurawat VJ, Finley JC, Galipeau PC, et al. Genetic mechanisms of TP53 loss of heterozygosity in Barrett's esophagus: implications for biomarker validation. Cancer Epidemiol Biomarkers Prev 2006;15:509–16.
40. Cestari R, Villanacci V, Rossi E, et al. Fluorescence in situ hybridization to evaluate dysplasia in Barrett's esophagus: a pilot study. Cancer Lett 2007;251: 278–87.
41. Rygiel AM, van Baal JW, Milano F, et al. Efficient automated assessment of genetic abnormalities detected by fluorescence in situ hybridization on brush cytology in a Barrett esophagus surveillance population. Cancer 2007;109: 1980–8.
42. Cawley HM, Meltzer SJ, De Benedetti VM, et al. Anti-p53 antibodies in patients with Barrett's esophagus or esophageal carcinoma can predate cancer diagnosis. Gastroenterology 1998;115:19–27.
43. Hetts SW. To die or not to die: an overview of apoptosis and its role in disease. JAMA 1998;279:300–7.
44. Shureiqi I, Xu X, Chen D, et al. Nonsteroidal anti-inflammatory drugs induce apoptosis in esophageal cancer cells by restoring 15-lipoxygenase-1 expression. Cancer Res 2001;61:4879–84.
45. Wilson KT, Fu S, Ramanujam KS, et al. Increased expression of inducible nitric oxide synthase and cyclooxygenase-2 in Barrett's esophagus and associated adenocarcinomas. Cancer Res 1998;58:2929–34.
46. Shirvani VN, Ouatu-Lascar R, Kaur BS, et al. Cyclooxygenase 2 expression in Barrett's esophagus and adenocarcinoma: ex vivo induction by bile salts and acid exposure. Gastroenterology 2000;118:487–96.

47. Suda T, Takahashi T, Golstein P, et al. Molecular cloning and expression of the Fas ligand, a novel member of the tumor necrosis factor family. Cell 1993;75:1169–78.
48. Younes M, Schwartz MR, Ertan A, et al. Fas ligand expression in esophageal carcinomas and their lymph node metastases. Cancer 2000;88:524–8.
49. Ferguson HR, Wild CP, Anderson LA, et al. Cyclooxygenase-2 and inducible nitric oxide synthase gene polymorphisms and risk of reflux esophagitis, Barrett's esophagus, and esophageal adenocarcinoma. Cancer Epidemiol Biomarkers Prev 2008;17:727–31.
50. Shay JW, Bacchetti S. A survey of telomerase activity in human cancer. Eur J Cancer 1997;33:787–91.
51. Morales CP, Lee EL, Shay JW. In situ hybridization for the detection of telomerase RNA in the progression from Barrett's esophagus to esophageal adenocarcinoma. Cancer 1998;83:652–9.
52. Lord RV, Salonga D, Danenberg KD, et al. Telomerase reverse transcriptase expression is increased early in the Barrett's metaplasia, dysplasia, adenocarcinoma sequence. J Gastrointest Surg 2000;4:135–42.
53. Barclay JY, Morris A, Nwokolo CU. Telomerase, hTERT and splice variants in Barrett's oesophagus and oesophageal adenocarcinoma. Eur J Gastroenterol Hepatol 2005;17:221–7.
54. Clement G, Braunschweig R, Pasquier N, et al. Methylation of APC, TIMP3, and TERT: a new predictive marker to distinguish Barrett's oesophagus patients at risk for malignant transformation. J Pathol 2006;208:100–7.
55. Auvinen MI, Sihvo EI, Ruohtula T, et al. Incipient angiogenesis in Barrett's epithelium and lymphangiogenesis in Barrett's adenocarcinoma. J Clin Oncol 2002;20:2971–9.
56. Achen MG, Jeltsch M, Kukk E, et al. Vascular endothelial growth factor D (VEGF-D) is a ligand for the tyrosine kinases VEGF receptor 2 (Flk1) and VEGF receptor 3 (Flt4). Proc Natl Acad Sci U S A 1998;95:548–53.
57. Lord RV, Park JM, Wickramasinghe K, et al. Vascular endothelial growth factor and basic fibroblast growth factor expression in esophageal adenocarcinoma and Barrett esophagus. J Thorac Cardiovasc Surg 2003;125:246–53.
58. Saad RS, El Gohary Y, Memari E, et al. Endoglin (CD105) and vascular endothelial growth factor as prognostic markers in esophageal adenocarcinoma. Hum Pathol 2005;36:955–61.
59. Bailey T, Biddlestone L, Shepherd N, et al. Altered cadherin and catenin complexes in the Barrett's esophagus-dysplasia-adenocarcinoma sequence: correlation with disease progression and dedifferentiation. Am J Pathol 1998;152:135–44.
60. Washington K, Chiappori A, Hamilton K, et al. Expression of beta-catenin, alpha-catenin, and E-cadherin in Barrett's esophagus and esophageal adenocarcinomas. Mod Pathol 1998;11:805–13.
61. Coussens LM, Fingleton B, Matrisian LM. Matrix metalloproteinase inhibitors and cancer: trials and tribulations. Science 2002;295:2387–92.
62. Herszenyi L, Hritz I, Pregun I, et al. Alterations of glutathione S-transferase and matrix metalloproteinase-9 expressions are early events in esophageal carcinogenesis. World J Gastroenterol 2007;13:676–82.
63. Murray GI, Duncan ME, O'Neil P, et al. Matrix metalloproteinase-1 is associated with poor prognosis in oesophageal cancer. J Pathol 1998;185:256–61.
64. Salmela MT, Karjalainen-Lindsberg ML, Puolakkainen P, et al. Upregulation and differential expression of matrilysin (MMP-7) and metalloelastase (MMP-12) and their inhibitors TIMP-1 and TIMP-3 in Barrett's oesophageal adenocarcinoma. Br J Cancer 2001;85:383–92.

65. Falkenback D, Nilbert M, Oberg S, et al. Prognostic value of cell adhesion in esophageal adenocarcinomas. Dis Esophagus 2008;21:97–102.
66. Osterheld MC, Bian YS, Bosman FT, et al. Beta-catenin expression and its association with prognostic factors in adenocarcinoma developed in Barrett esophagus. Am J Clin Pathol 2002;117:451–6.
67. Rabinovitch PS, Longton G, Blount PL, et al. Predictors of progression in Barrett's esophagus III: baseline flow cytometric variables. Am J Gastroenterol 2001;96: 3071–83.
68. Galipeau PC, Cowan DS, Sanchez CA, et al. 17p (p53) allelic losses, 4N (G2/tetraploid) populations, and progression to aneuploidy in Barrett's esophagus. Proc Natl Acad Sci U S A 1996;93:7081–4.
69. Kerkhof M, Steyerberg EW, Kusters JG, et al. Aneuploidy and high expression of p53 and Ki67 is associated with neoplastic progression in Barrett esophagus. Cancer Biomark 2008;4:1–10.
70. Rygiel AM, Milano F, Ten Kate FJ, et al. Assessment of chromosomal gains as compared to DNA content changes is more useful to detect dysplasia in Barrett's esophagus brush cytology specimens. Genes Chromosomes Cancer 2008;47: 396–404.
71. Pindur A, Chakraborty S, Welch DG, et al. DNA ploidy measurements in prostate cancer: differences between image analysis and flow cytometry and clinical implications. Prostate 1994;25:189–98.
72. Alanen KA, Lintu M, Joensuu H. Image cytometry of breast carcinomas that are DNA diploid by flow cytometry: time to revise the concept of DNA diploidy? Anal Quant Cytol Histol 1998;20:178–86.
73. Huang Q, Yu C, Zhang X, et al. Comparison of DNA histograms by standard flow cytometry and image cytometry on sections in Barrett's adenocarcinoma. BMC Clin Pathol 2008;8:5.
74. Shaheen NJ, Crosby MA, Bozymski EM, et al. Is there publication bias in the reporting of cancer risk in Barrett's esophagus? Gastroenterology 2000;119:333–8.
75. Daniely Y, Liao G, Dixon D, et al. Critical role of p63 in the development of a normal esophageal and tracheobronchial epithelium. Am J Physiol Cell Physiol 2004;287:C171–81.
76. Barker N, van Es JH, Kuipers J, et al. Identification of stem cells in small intestine and colon by marker gene Lgr5. Nature 2007;449:1003–7.
77. May R, Riehl TE, Hunt C, et al. Identification of a novel putative gastrointestinal stem cell and adenoma stem cell marker, doublecortin and CaM kinase-like-1, following radiation injury and in adenomatous polyposis coli/multiple intestinal neoplasia mice. Stem Cells 2008;26:630–7.
78. Adams JM, Strasser A. Is tumor growth sustained by rare cancer stem cells or dominant clones? Cancer Res 2008;68:4018–21.
79. Souza RF, Krishnan K, Spechler SJ. Acid, bile and CDX: the ABCs of making Barrett's metaplasia. Am J Physiol Gastrointest Liver Physiol 2008;295:G470–8.
80. Spechler SJ, Souza RF. Stem cells in Barrett's esophagus: HALOs or horns? Gastrointest Endosc 2008;68:41–3.

Risk Factors for Esophageal Cancer Development

Gary W. Falk, MD, MS

KEYWORDS

- Barrett's esophagus • Esophageal adenocarcinoma
- Cancer risk • Dysplasia • Gastroesophageal reflux disease

Adenocarcinoma of the esophagus was previously recognized as an uncommon disorder. Studies now show that the incidence of this cancer has increased by approximately six fold between 1975 and 2001, a rate greater than that of any other cancer in the United States during that time.[1] This increase has been accompanied by an increase in mortality rates from 2 to 15 deaths per million during that same time period. Similar findings are occurring elsewhere in the Western world today. The cause of this increase remains uncertain. This article explores the various risk factors for the development of esophageal adenocarcinoma (**Table 1**).

BARRETT'S ESOPHAGUS

Barrett's esophagus is a clearly recognized risk factor for the development of esophageal adenocarcinoma compared with the general population.[2] It is an acquired condition resulting from severe esophageal mucosal injury and is typically found in or adjacent to esophageal adenocarcinoma in resection specimens.[3] Cancer risk in Barrett's esophagus appears to be limited to patients with specialized columnar epithelium, although this concept has recently been questioned.

Despite the alarming increase in the incidence of esophageal adenocarcinoma, the precise incidence of adenocarcinoma in patients with Barrett's esophagus is uncertain, with rates varying from approximately 1/52 to 1/694 years of follow-up.[4] It is estimated that the risk of developing cancer in a given patient with Barrett's esophagus is approximately 0.5% to 0.7% annually with no clear evidence of geographic variation.[4,5] The evolving epidemiologic data suggest that despite the alarming increase in the incidence of esophageal adenocarcinoma, the vast majority of patients with Barrett's esophagus still will never develop cancer and will die of causes other than cancer.[6,7]

Department of Gastroenterology & Hepatology, Center for Swallowing and Esophageal Disorders, Desk A-31, Cleveland Clinic, 9500 Euclid Avenue, Cleveland, OH 44195, USA
E-mail address: falkg@ccf.org

Surg Oncol Clin N Am 18 (2009) 469–485
doi:10.1016/j.soc.2009.03.005
1055-3207/09/$ – see front matter © 2009 Elsevier Inc. All rights reserved.

surgonc.theclinics.com

Table 1
Risk factors for esophageal cancer and strength of association

Risk Factor	Strength of Association
Barrett's esophagus	+++
Dysplasia	+++
Segment length	±
Biomarkers of increased risk	+
Obesity	+++
Age	+++
Gender	+++
Race	+++
Reflux symptoms	++
Smoking	++
Family history	+
Diet	+
Alcohol consumption	±
H pylori infection	−
Aspirin/NSAID consumption	−
Vitamin consumption	−
Acid suppression	±
Antireflux surgery	±
Drugs that relax the LES	±

Strength of association: + = risk factor; − = protective factor; ± = equivocal or no clear evidence for or against.

The marked increase in the incidence of Barrett's esophagus was attributed by many to the increased use of diagnostic upper endoscopy combined with the change in the definition of Barrett's esophagus to include shorter segments of columnar-lined epithelium.[8] However, recent data from the Netherlands suggest that the incidence of Barrett's esophagus is in fact increasing in the general population independent of the number of upper endoscopies.[9]

A variety of characteristics of the Barrett's mucosa is associated with an increase in the risk for cancer.

Segment Length

Esophageal cancer develops in both short and long segments of Barrett's esophagus.[3] A variety of studies have examined if the risk of developing adenocarcinoma increases with increasing length of Barrett's epithelium. Intuitively, one would think that the greater the length, the greater the amount of mucosa at risk for cancer development. Studies to date have yielded mixed results for length as a risk factor, in part because of the low incidence of progression to cancer in cohort studies. Observational studies suggest that the prevalence of cancer and dysplasia is higher in longer lengths of Barrett's epithelium.[10–14] A prospective cohort study by Rudolph and colleagues[15] of the Seattle Barrett's Esophagus Research Program found that segment length was not related to subsequent risk of cancer. However, when subjects with high-grade dysplasia at index endoscopy were excluded, a nonsignificant trend for risk of cancer was noted. Weston and colleagues[13] found that a segment length of 6 cm or greater was associated with an increased risk for developing high-grade dysplasia or adeno-carcinoma. Others have also found an increased risk of subsequent development of dysplasia or carcinoma with increased length of Barrett's epithelium.[14,16] However, a recent meta-analysis found only a trend for decreased cancer risk for short-segment Barrett's esophagus.[4] Taken together, these data suggest that the relationship between segment length and cancer risk is uncertain.

Dysplasia

Barrett's esophagus patients progress through a phenotypic sequence of no dysplasia, low-grade dysplasia, high-grade dysplasia, and then adenocarcinoma, although the time course is highly variable and this stepwise sequence is not preor-dained.[17,18] Furthermore, some patients may progress directly to cancer without prior detection of dysplasia of any grade.[19] Currently, dysplasia remains the only factor useful for identifying patients at increased risk for the development of esophageal adenocarcinoma in clinical practice. Low-grade dysplasia is recognized adjacent to and distant from Barrett's esophagus–associated adenocarcinoma in resection spec-imens.[20,21] Furthermore, systematic esophagectomy-mapping studies demonstrate that low-grade dysplasia typically occupies a far greater surface area of the involved esophagus than does high-grade dysplasia or cancer.[21]

Low-grade dysplasia is characterized histologically by preserved crypt architecture, with abnormal nuclei in the basal half of the cell.[22] Despite that seemingly simple defi-nition, the diagnosis needs to be distinguished from reactive changes caused by inflammation or ulceration. Interobserver variability, even among expert GI patholo-gists in the interpretation of low-grade dysplasia, is especially problematic. Montgom-ery and colleagues[23] found interobserver agreement to be fair for low-grade dysplasia (kappa score of 0.32), but substantial for high-grade dysplasia or adenocarcinoma (kappa score of 0.65). The inability to reproducibly diagnose low-grade dysplasia may explain the highly variable natural history of this lesion.

What do we know about the natural history of low-grade dysplasia, given the limited number of subjects studied to date? First, the diagnosis is often transient,[24,25] which may be due in part to the high degree of interobserver variability in establishing this diagnosis and the variable biopsy protocols by which these subjects are followed, re-sulting in issues related to tissue sampling. While the majority of subjects with low-grade dysplasia do not progress to adenocarcinoma or high-grade dysplasia, a subset of these subjects do progress to a higher-grade lesion. Skacel and colleagues[26] fol-lowed 25 subjects with low-grade dysplasia for a mean of 26 months and found that 28% developed high-grade dysplasia or adenocarcinoma, whereas 60% regressed and 12% had persistent low-grade dysplasia. However, a consensus agreement among the GI pathologists in that study was associated with an increased risk for progression. Weston and colleagues[27] followed 48 subjects with low-grade dysplasia for a mean of 41 months and found that 10% progressed to multifocal high-grade dysplasia or adenocarcinoma, 65% regressed, and 25% had persistent low-grade dysplasia. More recently, a Veterans Affairs (VA) cohort study estimated that the risk for progressing to high-grade dysplasia or adenocarcinoma was 1.3%/year in subjects with baseline low-grade dysplasia compared with 0.36%/year in subjects without low-grade dysplasia.[28] However, a multicenter cohort study by Shar-ma and colleagues[19] identified 156 subjects with low-grade dysplasia, 13% of whom progressed to high-grade dysplasia or cancer for an incidence of 0.6%/year, a rate no different from most estimates for subjects with intestinal metaplasia without dysplasia.

Srivastava and colleagues[29] recently examined the significance of the extent of low-grade dysplasia as a risk factor for progression to cancer in 77 Barrett's esophagus subjects. They found that 31.8% of subjects with a maximum baseline diagnosis of low-grade dysplasia progressed to cancer compared with 68.2% of subjects with baseline high-grade dysplasia. In subjects with a maximum diagnosis of low-grade dysplasia at baseline, the mean proportion of low-grade crypts/subject was higher in progressors versus nonprogressors (64.5% versus 22.1%, $P = .01$). However, there was no relationship between extent (focal or diffuse) of low-grade dysplasia and cancer risk.

Thus, the natural history of low-grade dysplasia remains highly variable: some patients clearly progress to develop high-grade dysplasia or adenocarcinoma, whereas regression is seen in the majority of these individuals. However, "regression" in many cases could be related to diagnostic accuracy and/or sampling error. Taken together, studies to date suggest that low-grade dysplasia results in an intermediate risk for the development of adenocarcinoma.[30]

High-grade dysplasia in Barrett's esophagus is a well-recognized risk factor for the development of adenocarcinoma.[31–33] Unsuspected carcinoma is detected at esophagectomy in approximately 40% of patients with high-grade dysplasia, with a range of 0% to 73%.[34] Several recent studies have improved our understanding of the natural history of high-grade dysplasia. Buttar and colleagues[31] followed 100 subjects with high-grade dysplasia with continued endoscopic surveillance and found cancer at 1 and 3 years in 38% and 56% of individuals with diffuse high-grade dysplasia and 7% and 14% of individuals with focal high-grade dysplasia, respectively. Reid and colleagues[32] followed 76 subjects for five years and encountered cancer in 59%. On the other hand, Schnell and colleagues,[33] in a study of 79 subjects, found cancer in 5% of subjects during the first year of surveillance and in 16% of the remaining subjects followed for a mean of 7 years (20% of the total group developed cancer). Others have reported regression of high-grade dysplasia over time as well.[33,35] A recent meta-analysis found that the incidence of adenocarcinoma in subjects with high-grade dysplasia was approximately 6.58% annually.[36] Mucosal abnormalities in patients with multifocal high-grade dysplasia may also be a risk factor for adenocarcinoma.[31,37] Thus, high-grade dysplasia remains a worrisome lesion, although progression to carcinoma may take many years and is not inevitable.

Unfortunately, dysplasia is an imperfect marker of increased cancer risk. It is typically not distinguishable endoscopically and is often focal in nature, thereby making targeting of biopsies problematic. Furthermore, there is considerable interobserver variability in the grading of dysplasia in both the community and academic settings, and the ability of pathologists to distinguish between intramucosal carcinoma and high-grade dysplasia is problematic even in esophagectomy specimens.[23,38–40]

Biomarkers

A number of molecular markers may define patients at increased risk for the development of esophageal adenocarcinoma. Among the most frequently described molecular changes that precede the development of adenocarcinoma in Barrett's esophagus are alterations in p53 (mutation, deletion, or loss of heterozygosity [LOH]);[41–44] p16 (mutation, deletion, promoter hypermethylation, or LOH);[41,45–47] and aneuploidy by flow cytometry.[48,49] Neoplastic progression in Barrett's esophagus is accompanied by flow cytometric abnormalities such as aneuploidy or increased G2/tetraploid DNA contents, and these abnormalities may precede the development of high-grade dysplasia or adenocarcinoma.[48,49] The potential importance of flow cytometry as a prognostic biomarker was illustrated in work by Reid and colleagues,[32] who found that for subjects with no flow cytometric abnormalities at baseline and with histology that showed no dysplasia, indefinite or low-grade dysplasia, the five-year incidence of cancer was 0%. In contrast, aneuploidy, increased 4N fractions, or high-grade dysplasia was detected in each of the 35 subjects who went on to develop cancer within five years.

Mutations of p53 and 17p LOH have been reported in up to 92% and 100%, respectively, of esophageal adenococarcinomas.[43] Furthermore, both abnormalities have been detected in Barrett's epithelium before the development of carcinoma.[42–44] For example, Reid and colleagues[42] found that the prevalence of 17p (p53) LOH at baseline increased from 6% in subjects negative for dysplasia to 20% in subjects with low-grade dysplasia, and to 57% in subjects with high-grade dysplasia. More importantly, the 3-year incidence of cancer was 38% for individuals with 17p (p53) LOH compared with 3.3% for individuals with two 17p alleles. However, techniques to detect p53 mutations and 17p LOH are labor intensive and have not achieved widespread acceptance in clinical practice to date. Similarly, p16 LOH and inactivation of the p16 gene by promoter region hypermethylation have been reported frequently in esophageal adenocarcinoma.[47] Furthermore, 9p LOH is commonly encountered in premalignant Barrett's epithelium and can be detected over large regions of the Barrett's mucosa.[47] It is hypothesized that clonal expansion occurs in conjunction with p16 abnormalities, creating a field in which other genetic lesions leading to esophageal adenocarcinoma can arise.

Epigenetic changes, in the form of hypo- and hypermethylation and alteration to histone complexes have also been implicated in the progression of Barrett's esophagus to adenocarcinoma. Hypermethylation of p16, RUNX3, and HPP1 are all independently associated with an increased risk of progression of Barrett's esophagus to high-grade dysplasia or esophageal adenocarcinoma.[50]

Given the complexity and diversity of alterations observed to date in the metaplasia, dysplasia, carcinoma sequence, it appears that a panel of biomarkers may be required for risk stratification. Two recent studies have examined just such an approach with promising results. The combination of 17p LOH, 9p LOH, and DNA-content abnormality has been shown to predict the 10-year adenocarcinoma risk better than any single biomarker alone. Subjects with a combination of these abnormalities had a markedly increased risk of developing cancer compared with those with no baseline abnormalities (relative risk 38.7; 95% CI, 10.8–138.5). In those with no abnormalities of any of these biomarkers at baseline, 12% developed adenocarcinoma at 10 years. In contrast, those with the combination of 17p LOH, 9p LOH, and DNA-content abnormality had a cumulative incidence of adenocarcinoma of 79% over the same period.[51] A risk stratification model using a methylation index constructed from the methylation values for p16, HPP1, and RUNX3 also showed potential for prediction of progression to high-grade dysplasia or adenocarcinoma.[52] All of these studies demonstrate the potential for biomarkers to predict risk of esophageal adenocarcinoma. Unfortunately, none of these biomarkers have been validated in large-scale clinical trials to date and as such are not yet useful for clinical decision making.

REFLUX SYMPTOMS AND ESOPHAGITIS

Two studies have examined the relationship between esophagitis and esophageal adenocarcinoma. Solaymani-Dodaran and colleagues,[2] using the General Practice Research Database in the United Kingdom, found that the relative risk for esophageal adenocarcinoma was elevated to 4.5 (95% CI, 1.04–19.6) among esophagitis subjects compared with the general population. Subsequently, a Danish population-based cohort study found that the standardized incidence ratio for esophageal adenocarcinoma was elevated to 5.38 (95% CI, 3.01–8.87) among subjects with esophagitis.[53]

However, 10 of the 15 subjects who developed esophageal adenocarcinoma in that study had Barrett's esophagus diagnosed at least one year before discovery of the cancer suggesting that most of the cancers were related to Barrett's esophagus and not esophagitis per se.

What about GERD symptoms alone? The General Practice Research Database study of Solaymani-Dodaran found no relationship between subjects with a prior diagnosis of GERD without esophagitis and subsequent risk of developing esophageal adenocarcinoma.[2] On the other hand, the landmark case-control Swedish population-based study by Lagergren and colleagues[54] found that the more severe, frequent, and persistent the symptoms of reflux, the greater the risk of esophageal adenocarcinoma. However, this work and that of others has shown that approximately 40% of subjects with esophageal adenocarcinoma have no history of regular reflux symptoms.[54,55]

AGE

Studies consistently show that the incidence of esophageal adenocarcinoma increases with age. Data from both the Surveillance, Epidemiology, and End Results (SEER) program and the Danish Cancer Registry demonstrate that the incidence rate of esophageal adenocarcinoma increases with age until it peaks at 75–79 years of age and declines thereafter.[56,57] Furthermore, El-Serag and colleagues,[56] using the SEER database, observed that this age effect has shifted upwards with time, as there has been an increase in the incidence of esophageal adenocarcinoma among younger subjects in addition to the older age groups. This suggests a cohort effect, with higher incidence rates seen among cohorts of subjects born most recently. El-Serag calculated that the odds of developing esophageal adenocarcinoma increased by 6.6% for each 5–year increase in age. (OR 1.066, 95% CI, 1.060–1.072)

GENDER

Male gender is a well-recognized risk factor for esophageal adenocarcinoma. It is estimated that the incidence of esophageal adenocarcinoma is approximately six to eight fold greater in men than in women.[56,57] That being said, the incidence of esophageal adenocarcinoma is increasing steadily in both genders.

RACE

White race has long been associated with esophageal adenocarcinoma.[56,58–60] A recent analysis of SEER cancer registry data from 1992 through 1998 provided the most comprehensive analysis of the role of ethnicity in esophageal cancer to date. Kubo and Corley[61] found that the average annual incidence rate for esophageal adenocarcinoma for white men was double that of Hispanic men (4.2 versus 2.0/100,000/year). This rate was also four times higher than that seen in blacks, Asians/Pacific Islanders and Native Americans. Similar patterns were seen in women, where the rates for all ethnicities were lower than that encountered among the men. Interestingly, the incidence rates for esophageal adenocarcinoma increased only for the white population between 1992 and 1998 but not for the other ethnic groups. Thus, there are clear ethnic imbalances in the risk for esophageal adenocarcinoma.

FAMILY HISTORY

Given the clear association of esophageal adenocarcinoma with male gender and white race, a possible inherited component to the risk of esophageal carcinoma has long been hypothesized. This hypothesis has been supported by a number of reports of familial clustering of both Barrett's esophagus and esophageal adenocarcinoma.[62–66] These small studies suggest the possibility of an autosomal dominant inheritance pattern. Larger case-control studies come to less clear-cut conclusions. First, a population-based case-control study in the United States found no association between the risk of esophageal adenocarcinoma and a family history of digestive disease cancers either as a group or by individual sites.[67] Two Swedish case-control studies came to different conclusions. Lagergren and colleagues[68] found that the occurrence of esophageal cancer of any histology among first-degree relatives did not increase the risk of esophageal adenocarcinoma. In contrast, Ji and colleagues,[69] using an updated version of the Swedish Family Cancer Database, found that the standardized incidence ratio for esophageal adenocarcinoma (observed: expected cases) was elevated to 3.52 (95% CI, 1.11–8.28) among offspring of parents with esophageal cancer of any subtype. However, if the parental proband had esophageal adenocarcinoma, the subsequent risk of adenocarcinoma in offspring was not increased. However, none of the affected parents were diagnosed with esophageal adenocarcinoma. Finally, Chak and colleagues[70] found that a positive family history was higher among cases with Barrett's esophagus, esophageal adenocarcinoma, or gastroesophageal junction adenocarcinoma than among GERD controls (24% versus 5%). The familial effect was present in all three of the subgroups studied. Taken together, these studies suggest that inherited factors may represent a risk factor for the development of esophageal adenocarcinoma in a small subset of subjects. The exact magnitude of the risk and the gene(s) associated with this risk are currently under investigation.

OBESITY

The rapid increase in the incidence of esophageal adenocarcinoma has paralleled the rise of obesity in the Western world. As such, obesity has emerged as a leading candidate risk factor for esophageal adenocarcinoma. A variety of observational studies have demonstrated a relationship between obesity and esophageal adenocarcinoma. A number of studies have also demonstrated an association between increasing BMI and increased risk of esophageal adenocarcinoma.[71–76] Several systematic reviews and meta-analyses have confirmed these observations.[77,78] Kubo and Corley[78] found that a BMI greater than 25 was associated with an increased risk of esophageal adenocarcinoma in both men (OR 2.2; 85% CI, 1.7–2.7) and women (OR 2.0; 95% CI, 1.4–2.9) and higher levels of BMI were associated with increased risk.

Recent studies have helped to fine tune our understanding of the association between obesity and esophageal adenocarcinoma risk. A population-based case-control study from Australia found that obesity increased the risk of esophageal adenocarcinoma in a dose-dependent fashion, with the highest risk encountered for a BMI of 40 kg/m^2 or greater when compared with a healthy BMI.[79] Furthermore, risks associated with obesity were noted to be higher in men than in women. Corley and colleagues[80] extended these observations and examined the distribution of obesity and cancer risk in a case-control study. They found that increasing abdominal diameter was strongly associated with an increased risk of esophageal adenocarcinoma in a dose-dependent manner, which did not change when adjusted for BMI (OR 4.78; 95% CI, 1.14–20.11). The fact that abdominal obesity is more common among men could also explain the male predilection for this cancer.

Is there a mechanism that could explain the association of obesity and cancer risk? Obesity, especially central obesity, increases intragastric pressure and the gastroesophageal pressure gradient, thereby facilitating reflux of contents into the esophagus. This increase in pressure gradient is accompanied by a predisposition for hiatal hernia, another risk factor for the development of reflux and complications such as Barrett's esophagus.[81] Metabolic effects of obesity, especially abdominal obesity, may also contribute to these observations. A variety of hormones, including leptin, adiponectin, insulin-like growth factors, insulin, and sex steroids are associated with increasing adiposity.[82] These hormones modulate cellular proliferation and apoptosis, thereby providing biologic plausibility for the relationship of obesity and carcinogenesis independent of reflux.

HELICOBACTER PYLORI

The prevalence of H pylori infection has been falling in the Western world at the same time that the incidence of esophageal carcinoma has been increasing.[83] Thus it is natural to look for a relationship between these two opposing time trends. A number of epidemiologic studies have demonstrated a negative association between H pylori infection and esophageal adenocarcinoma.[84–87] This association has also been described with the cagA+ strain, which is felt to result in more intense inflammation and a greater tendency to gastric atrophy.[86–88] A recent meta-analysis found the pooled odds ratio for the prevalence of H pylori infection in esophageal adenocarcinoma to be 0.52 (95% CI, 0.37–0.73) and for the H pylori cagA+ strain to be 0.51 (95% CI, 0.31–0.82).[89]

The primary mechanism postulated for this protective effect centers around decreased acid secretion caused by H pylori induced gastric atrophy, especially with cagA+ strains.[83] A recent population-based case-control study from Ireland found that severe gastric atrophy, as measured by pepsinogen I/II ratios, was associated with a clearly decreased risk of esophageal adenocarcinoma, giving support to this as a putative mechanism of protection from esophageal adenocarcinoma. However, that same study also found the protective effect of H pylori infection was also encountered in atrophy-negative subjects, suggesting that mechanisms other than gastric atrophy are involved in the potential protective effects of H pylori infection for esophageal adenocarcinoma, such as neutralization of acid by ammonia produced by H pylori, proapoptotic effects of H pylori on adenocarcinoma cell lines, and alterations in ghrelin secretion.[83]

SMOKING

A number of studies have identified current or past smoking as a risk factor for esophageal adenocarcinoma.[74,90–96] The risk increases with increasing intensity and duration of smoking.[94,95] Interestingly, the risk associated with smoking persists with little reduction of risk observed until 30 years after smoking cessation.[94] However, a Swedish population-based case-control study did not identify smoking as a risk factor for esophageal adenocarcinoma.[97]

ALCOHOL CONSUMPTION

Most epidemiologic studies find no association between alcohol consumption and esophageal adenocarcinoma.[90–92,94,95,97,98] However, several studies do find a modest association of alcohol consumption and risk of esophageal adenocarcinoma.[93,96] Taken together, alcohol consumption does not appear to be a major risk factor for esophageal adenocarcinoma.

DIET

A variety of studies have examined diet and food supplements and risk of esophageal adenocarcinoma. Increased consumption of fruits and vegetables is consistently associated with a decrease in the risk for esophageal adenocarcinoma.[99–102] In fact, Engel and colleagues[99] found that the population attributable risk, defined as the proportion of a disease in the population attributable to a given risk factor, associated with low consumption of fruits and vegetables was 15.3% (95% CI, 5.8%–34.6%). At the same time, higher intake of saturated fats and red meat may increase cancer risk.[100,101]

A diet high in carbohydrates may be linked to cancer.[103] A recent ecologic study found a correlation between the rise in carbohydrate consumption with the increase in esophageal adenocarcinoma rates.[103] While ecologic studies should be viewed as hypothesis generating, and are flawed by the concept of ecologic fallacy, this observation is in fact plausible. A high carbohydrate diet can lead to insulin resistance, and hence elevated levels of both insulin and insulin-like growth factor, both of which have been implicated in carcinogenesis. Despite increasing attention, there does not seem to be an association between carbonated drink consumption and risk of esophageal adenocarcinoma.[104,105]

Lastly, the role of dietary supplements and esophageal adenocarcinoma has also been examined by a number of investigators. Recent work from the Seattle Barrett's Esophagus Research Program found that consumption of one or more multivitamins daily was associated with a decrease in the hazard ratio of developing esophageal adenocarcinoma (HR 0.38, 95% CI, 0.15–0.99) compared with subjects not taking multivitamins.[106] Similar findings were encountered for daily use of vitamins C and E in that same study. Others have also found a reduced risk of esophageal adenocarcinoma associated with antioxidant vitamin consumption.[107]

NSAIDS AND ASPIRIN

A number of observational studies suggest that NSAIDs, including aspirin, may play a protective role against esophageal adenocarcinoma by inhibiting the cycloxygenase 1 and 2 enzymes, which regulate PGE2 production.[108–113] One possible mechanism that is involved in reflux-associated carcinogenesis in Barrett's esophagus is acid and bile salt induced COX-2 activation and high levels of PGE2 production. A systematic review suggested that the protective effect of aspirin and NSAIDs was greater with more regular use, an observation supported in a recent cohort study as well.[108,111] However, others could find no protective effect for esophageal cancer with long-term use of NSAIDs.[114]

A single clinical trial examined the effect of celecoxib at a dose of 200 mg twice daily given for 48 weeks in subjects with low-grade and high-grade dysplasia on change in proportion of biopsy samples with dysplasia between subjects treated with celecoxib compared with those treated with a placebo.[115] No differences were found between the two groups. A small crossover study demonstrated that high-dose PPI therapy in conjunction with aspirin at a dose of 325 mg daily can decrease mucosal PGE-2 content in mucosal biopsies from Barrett's esophagus subjects.[116] These findings led to a large randomized clinical trial in the United Kingdom (ASPECT) and a smaller clinical trial in the United States in an effort to examine the potential for chemoprevention with aspirin in conjunction with a proton pump inhibitor as a clinical strategy in Barrett's esophagus patients.

ACID SUPPRESSION

Because Barrett's esophagus has the most severe pathophysiologic abnormalities of GERD, it should come as no surprise that proton pump inhibitors (PPIs) are the cornerstone of medical therapy for Barrett's esophagus. A recent VA cohort study suggested that PPI therapy, especially long-duration use, was associated with a decreased risk for the development of dysplasia.[117] However, most of the cases of dysplasia were low-grade, a lesion with an intermediate and highly variable risk for development of cancer. Similar observational data on reduction of dysplasia risk with administration of PPIs have been obtained in Australia.[118] However, there are no randomized controlled trials that have examined the issue of dysplasia or cancer prevention and administration of PPI therapy.

ANTIREFLUX SURGERY

Some have hypothesized that antireflux surgery provides protection from progression of Barrett's esophagus to adenocarcinoma.[119] However two lines of evidence suggest that antireflux surgery does not protect patients from developing esophageal adenocarcinoma. A large population-based cohort study from Sweden of GERD subjects found no protective effect for surgery.[120] The standardized incidence ratio of esophageal adenocarcinoma in the surgically treated group was 14.1, 95% CI, 8.0–22.8 compared with 6.3, 95% CI, 4.5–8.7 in the medically treated group. A VA cohort study also found no attenuation of the risk for developing esophageal adenocarcinoma in surgically treated compared with medically treated GERD subjects (0.072%/year versus 0.04%/year).[121]

Similar findings are seen in Barrett's esophagus patients. A meta-analysis of surgical versus medical therapy of Barrett's esophagus found no difference in the risk of esophageal adenocarcinoma between the two groups.[122] A subsequent systematic review by Chang and colleagues[123] found no difference in the incidence of esophageal adenocarcinoma in medically versus surgically treated subjects, and that any evidence suggesting otherwise was driven by uncontrolled case series. Thus, the best available evidence suggests that antireflux surgery does not decrease cancer risk in GERD or Barrett's esophagus patients.

DRUGS THAT RELAX THE LOWER ESOPHAGEAL SPHINCTER

The Swedish population-based case-control study of Lagergren and colleagues[124] found a positive association between medications that relax the lower esophageal sphincter and esophageal adenocarcinoma. However, this association disappeared after adjustment for reflux symptoms, suggesting that promotion of reflux was the cause of this observation. However, Vaughan and colleagues[125] found no such association in a population-based case-control study in the United States.

SUMMARY

The increase in the incidence of esophageal adenocarcinoma is alarming. It is clear that Barrett's esophagus is the single best identified risk factor for the development of esophageal adenocarcinoma, yet the overwhelming majority of Barrett's patients will never develop this cancer. It appears that the current epidemic of obesity is a major risk factor for the development of esophageal adenocarcinoma, perhaps in conjunction with both a decline in the prevalence of H pylori infection and the overall aging of the population in the Western world. A better understanding of exposures that increase and decrease risk of esophageal adenocarcinoma is urgently needed if this disturbing trend in cancer incidence is to be reversed.

REFERENCES

1. Pohl H, Welch HG. The role of overdiagnosis and reclassification in the marked increase of esophageal adenocarcinoma incidence. J Natl Cancer Inst 2005;97: 142–6.
2. Solaymani-Dodaran M, Logan RF, West J, et al. Risk of oesophageal cancer in Barrett's oesophagus and gastro-oesophageal reflux. Gut 2004;53:1070–4.
3. Cameron AJ, Lomboy CT, Pera M, et al. Adenocarcinoma of the esophagogastric junction and Barrett's esophagus. Gastroenterology 1995;109:1541–6.
4. Thomas T, Abrams KR, De Caestecker JS, et al. Meta analysis: cancer risk in Barrett's oesophagus. Aliment Pharmacol Ther 2007;26:1465–77.
5. Shaheen NJ, Crosby MA, Bozymski EM, et al. Is there publication bias in the reporting of cancer risk in Barrett's esophagus? Gastroenterology 2000;119: 333–8.
6. Moayyedi P, Burch N, Akhtar-Danesh N, et al. Mortality rates in patients with Barrett's oesophagus. Aliment Pharmacol Ther 2008;27:316–20.
7. van der Burgh A, Dees J, Hop WC, et al. Oesophageal cancer is an uncommon cause of death in patients with Barrett's oesophagus. Gut 1996;39:5–8.
8. Conio M, Cameron AJ, Romero Y, et al. Secular trends in the epidemiology and outcome of Barrett's oesophagus in Olmsted County, Minnesota. Gut 2001;48: 304–9.
9. van Soest EM, Dieleman JP, Siersema PD, et al. Increasing incidence of Barrett's oesophagus in the general population. Gut 2005;54:1062–6.
10. Weston AP, Krmpotich PT, Cherian R, et al. Prospective long-term endoscopic and histological follow-up of short segment Barrett's esophagus: comparison with traditional long segment Barrett's esophagus. Am J Gastroenterol 1997; 92:407–13.
11. Hirota WK, Loughney TM, Lazas DJ, et al. Specialized intestinal metaplasia, dysplasia, and cancer of the esophagus and esophagogastric junction: prevalence and clinical data. Gastroenterology 1999;116:277–85.
12. Avidan B, Sonnenberg A, Schnell TG, et al. Hiatal hernia size, Barrett's length, and severity of acid reflux are all risk factors for esophageal adenocarcinoma. Am J Gastroenterol 2002;97:1930–6.
13. Weston AP, Sharma P, Mathur S, et al. Risk stratification of Barrett's esophagus: updated prospective multivariate analysis. Am J Gastroenterol 2004;99: 1657–66.
14. Gopal DV, Lieberman DA, Magaret N, et al. Risk factors for dysplasia in patients with Barrett's esophagus (BE): results from a multicenter consortium. Dig Dis Sci 2003;48:1537–41.
15. Rudolph RE, Vaughan TL, Storer BE, et al. Effect of segment length on risk for neoplastic progression in patients with Barrett esophagus. Ann Intern Med 2000;132:612–20.
16. Hage M, Siersema PD, van Dekken H, et al. Oesophageal cancer incidence and mortality in patients with long-segment Barrett's oesophagus after a mean follow-up of 12.7 years. Scand J Gastroenterol 2004;39:1175–9.
17. Van Sandick JW, Van Lanschot JJ, Kuiken BW, et al. Impact of endoscopic biopsy surveillance of Barrett's esophagus on pathological stage and clinical outcome of Barrett's carcinoma. Gut 1998;43:216–22.

18. Hameeteman W, Tytgat GN, Houthoff HJ, et al. Barrett's esophagus: development of dysplasia and adenocarcinoma. Gastroenterology 1989;96:1249–56.

19. Sharma P, Falk GW, Weston AP, et al. Dysplasia and cancer in a large multi-center cohort of patients with Barrett's esophagus. Clin Gastroenterol Hepatol 2006;4:566–72.

20. McArdle JE, Lewin KJ, Randall G, et al. Distribution of dysplasias and early invasive carcinoma in Barrett's esophagus. Hum Pathol 1992;23:479–82.

21. Cameron AJ, Carpenter HA. Barrett's esophagus, high-grade dysplasia, and early adenocarcinoma: a pathological study. Am J Gastroenterol 1997;92:586–91.

22. Haggitt RC. Barrett's esophagus, dysplasia, and adenocarcinoma. Hum Pathol 1994;25:982–93.

23. Montgomery E, Bronner MP, Goldblum JR, et al. Reproducibility of the diagnosis of dysplasia in Barrett's esophagus: a reaffirmation. Hum Pathol 2001;32:368–78.

24. Offman JJ, Lewin K, Ramers C, et al. The economic impact of the diagnosis of dysplasia in Barrett's esophagus. Am J Gastroenterol 2000;95:2946–52.

25. Conio M, Blanchi S, Lapertosa G, et al. Long-term endoscopic surveillance of patients with Barrett's esophagus. Incidence of dysplasia and adenocarcinoma: a prospective study. Am J Gastroenterol 2003;98:1931–9.

26. Skacel M, Petras RE, Gramlich TL, et al. The diagnosis of low-grade dysplasia in Barrett's esophagus and its implications for disease progression. Am J Gastroenterol 2000;95:3383–7.

27. Weston AP, Banerjee SK, Sharma P, et al. p53 protein overexpression in low-grade dysplasia (LGD) in Barrett's esophagus: immunohistochemical marker predictive of progression. Am J Gastroenterol 2001;96:1355–62.

28. Dulai GS, Shekelle PG, Jensen DM, et al. Dysplasia and risk of further neoplastic progression in a regional veterans administration Barrett's cohort. Am J Gastroenterol 2005;100:775–83.

29. Srivastava A, Hornick JL, Li X, et al. Extent of low-grade dysplasia is a risk factor for the development of esophageal adenocarcinoma in Barrett's esophagus. Am J Gastroenterol 2007;102:483–93.

30. Sharma P. Low-grade dysplasia in Barrett's esophagus. Gastroenterology 2004;127:1233–8.

31. Buttar NS, Wang KK, Sebo TJ, et al. Extent of high-grade dysplasia in Barrett's esophagus correlates with risk of adenocarcinoma. Gastroenterology 2001;120:1630–9.

32. Reid BJ, Levine DS, Longton G, et al. Predictors of progression to cancer in Barrett's esophagus: baseline histology and flow cytometry identify low- and high-risk patient subsets. Am J Gastroenterol 2000;95:1669–76.

33. Schnell TG, Sontag SJ, Chejfec G, et al. Long-term nonsurgical management of Barrett's esophagus with high-grade dysplasia. Gastroenterology 2001;120:1607–19.

34. Pellegrini CA, Pohl D. High-grade dysplasia in Barrett's esophagus: surveillance or operation? J Gastrointest Surg 2000;4:131–4.

35. Weston AP, Sharma P, Topalovski M, et al. Long-term follow-up of Barrett's high-grade dysplasia. Am J Gastroenterol 2000;95:1888–93.

36. Rastogi A, Puli S, El-Serag HB, et al. Incidence of esophageal adenocarcinoma in patients with Barrett's esophagus and high-grade dysplasia: a meta-analysis. Gastrointest Endosc 2008;67:394–8.

37. Tharavej C, Hagen JA, Peters JH, et al. Predictive factors of coexisting cancer in Barrett's high-grade dysplasia. Surg Endosc 2006;20:439–43.

38. Alikhan M, Rex D, Khan A, et al. Variable pathologic interpretation of columnar lined esophagus by general pathologists in community practice. Gastrointest Endosc 1999;50:23–6.
39. Reid BJ, Haggitt RC, Rubin CE. Observer variation in the diagnosis of dysplasia in Barrett's esophagus. Hum Pathol 1988;19:166–78.
40. Ormsby AH, Petras RE, Henricks WH, et al. Observer variation in the diagnosis of superficial oesophageal adenocarcinoma. Gut 2002;51:671–6.
41. Galipeau PC, Prevo LJ, Sanchez CA, et al. Clonal expansion and loss of heterozygosity at chromosomes 9p and 17p in premalignant esophageal (Barrett's) tissue. J Natl Cancer Inst 1999;91:2087–95.
42. Reid BJ, Prevo LJ, Galipeau PC, et al. Predictors of progression in Barrett's esophagus II: baseline 17p (p53) loss of heterozygosity identifies a patient subset at increased risk for neoplastic progression. Am J Gastroenterol 2001; 96:2839–48.
43. Reid BJ. P53 and neoplastic progression in Barrett's esophagus. Am J Gastroenterol 2001;96:1321–3.
44. Prevo LJ, Sanchez CA, Galipeau PC, et al. Reid BJ P53-mutant clones and field effects in Barrett's esophagus. Cancer Res 1999;59:4784–7.
45. Wong DJ, Barrett MT, Stoger R, et al. p16INK4a promoter is hypermethylated at a high frequency in esophageal adenocarcinomas. Cancer Res 1997;57: 2619–22.
46. Bian YS, Osterheld MC, Fontolliet C, et al. P16 inactivation by methylation of the CDKN2A promoter occurs early during neoplastic progression in Barrett's esophagus. Gastroenterology 2002;122:1113–21.
47. Wong DJ, Paulson TG, Prevo LJ, et al. p16INK4a lesions are common, early abnormalities that undergo clonal expansion in Barrett's metaplastic epithelium. Cancer Res 2001;61:8284–9.
48. Reid BJ, Haggitt RC, Rubin CE, et al. Barrett's esophagus. Correlation between flow cytometry and histology in detection of patients at risk for adenocarcinoma. Gastroenterology 1987;93:1–11.
49. Reid BJ, Blount PL, Rubin CE, et al. Flow-cytometric and histological progression to malignancy in Barrett's esophagus: prospective endoscopic surveillance of a cohort. Gastroenterology 1992;102:1212–9.
50. Schulmann K, Sterian A, Berki A, et al. Inactivation of p16, RUNX3, and HPP1 occurs early in Barrett's-associated neoplastic progression and predicts progression risk. Oncogene 2005;24:4138–48.
51. Galipeau PC, Li X, Blount PL, et al. NSAIDs modulate CDKN2A, TP53, and DNA content risk for progression to esophageal adenocarcinoma. PLoS Med 2007;4: e67.
52. Sato F, Jin Z, Schulmann K, et al. Three-tiered risk stratification model to predict progression in Barrett's esophagus using epigenetic and clinical features. PLoS ONE 2008;3:e1890.
53. Lassen A, Hallas J, de Muckadell OB. Esophagitis: incidence and risk of esophageal adenocarcinoma–a population-based cohort study. Am J Gastroenterol 2006;101:1193–9.
54. Lagergren J, Bergström R, Lindgren A, et al. Symptomatic gastroesophageal reflux as a risk factor for esophageal adenocarcinoma. N Engl J Med 1999; 340:825–31.
55. Chak A, Faulx A, Eng C, et al. Gastroesophageal reflux symptoms in patients with adenocarcinoma of the esophagus or cardia. Cancer 2006; 107:2160–6.

56. El-Serag HB, Mason AC, Petersen N, et al. Epidemiological differences between adenocarcinoma of the oesophagus and adenocarcinoma of the gastric cardia in the USA. Gut 2002;50:368–72.
57. van Blankenstein M, Looman CW, Hop WC, et al. The incidence of adenocarcinoma and squamous cell carcinoma of the esophagus: Barrett's esophagus makes a difference. Am J Gastroenterol 2005;100:766–74.
58. Rogers EL, Goldkind SF, Iseri OA, et al. Adenocarcinoma of the lower esophagus. A disease primarily of white men with Barrett's esophagus. J Clin Gastroenterol 1986;8:613–8.
59. Chalasani N, Wo JM, Waring JP. Racial differences in the histology, location, and risk factors of esophageal cancer. J Clin Gastroenterol 1998;26:11–3.
60. Younes M, Henson DE, Ertan A, et al. Incidence and survival trends of esophageal carcinoma in the United States: racial and gender differences by histological type. Scand J Gastroenterol 2002;37:1359–65.
61. Kubo A, Corley DA. Marked multi-ethnic variation of esophageal and gastric cardia carcinomas within the United States. Am J Gastroenterol 2004;99:582–8.
62. Crabb DW, Berk MA, Hall TR, et al. Familial gastroesophageal reflux and development of Barrett's esophagus. Ann Intern Med 1985;103:52–4.
63. Jochem VJ, Fuerst PA, Fromkes JJ. Familial Barrett's esophagus associated with adenocarcinoma. Gastroenterology 1992;102:1400–2.
64. Fahmy N, King JF. Barrett's esophagus: an acquired condition with genetic predisposition. Am J Gastroenterol 1993;88:1262–5.
65. Eng C, Spechler SJ, Ruben R, et al. Familial Barrett esophagus and adenocarcinoma of the gastroesophageal junction. Cancer Epidemiol Biomarkers Prev 1993;2:397–9.
66. Poynton AR, Walsh TN, O'Sullivan G, et al. Carcinoma arising in familial Barrett's esophagus. Am J Gastroenterol 1996;91:1855–6.
67. Dhillon PK, Farrow DC, Vaughan TL, et al. Family history of cancer and risk of esophageal and gastric cancers in the United States. Int J Cancer 2001;93:148–52.
68. Lagergren J, Ye W, Lindgren A, et al. Heredity and risk of cancer of the esophagus and gastric cardia. Cancer Epidemiol Biomarkers Prev 2000;9:757–60.
69. Ji J, Hemminki K. Familial risk for esophageal cancer: an updated epidemiologic study from Sweden. Clin Gastroenterol Hepatol 2006;4:840–5.
70. Chak A, Lee T, Kinnard MF, et al. Familial aggregation of Barrett's oesophagus, oesophageal adenocarcinoma, and oesophagogastric junctional adenocarcinoma in Caucasian adults. Gut 2002;51:323–8.
71. Abnet CC, Freedman ND, Hollenbeck AR, et al. A prospective study of BMI and risk of oesophageal and gastric adenocarcinoma. Eur J Cancer 2008;44:465–71.
72. Merry AH, Schouten LJ, Goldbohm RA, et al. Body mass index, height and risk of adenocarcinoma of the oesophagus and gastric cardia: a prospective cohort study. Gut 2007;56:1503–11.
73. Engeland A, Tretli S, Bjørge T. Height and body mass index in relation to esophageal cancer; 23-year follow-up of two million Norwegian men and women. Cancer Causes Control 2004;15:837–43.
74. Veugelers PJ, Porter GA, Guernsey DL, et al. Obesity and lifestyle risk factors for gastroesophageal reflux disease, Barrett esophagus and esophageal adenocarcinoma. Dis Esophagus 2006;19:321–8.
75. Lagergren J, Bergström R, Nyrén O. Association between body mass and adenocarcinoma of the esophagus and gastric cardia. Ann Intern Med 1999;130:883–90.

76. Chow WH, Blot WJ, Vaughan TL, et al. Body mass index and risk of adenocarcinomas of the esophagus and gastric cardia. J Natl Cancer Inst 1998;90:150–5.
77. Hampel H, Abraham NS, El-Serag HB. Meta-analysis: obesity and the risk for gastroesophageal reflux disease and its complications. Ann Intern Med 2005; 143:199–211.
78. Kubo A, Corley DA. Body mass index and adenocarcinomas of the esophagus or gastric cardia: a systematic review and meta-analysis. Cancer Epidemiol Biomarkers Prev 2006;15:872–8.
79. Whiteman DC, Sadeghi S, Pandeya N, et al. Australian Cancer Study. Combined effects of obesity, acid reflux and smoking on the risk of adenocarcinomas of the oesophagus. Gut 2008;57:173–80.
80. Corley DA, Kubo A, Zhao W. Abdominal obesity and the risk of esophageal and gastric cardia carcinomas. Cancer Epidemiol Biomarkers Prev 2008;17:352–8.
81. Pandolfino JE, El-Serag HB, Zhang Q, et al. Obesity: a challenge to esophagogastric junction integrity. Gastroenterology 2006;130:639–49.
82. Moayyedi P. Barrett's esophagus and obesity: the missing part of the puzzle. Am J Gastroenterol 2008;103:301–3.
83. McColl KE, Watabe H, Derakhshan MH. Role of gastric atrophy in mediating negative association between *Helicobacter pylori* infection and reflux oesophagitis, Barrett's oesophagus and oesophageal adenocarcinoma. Gut 2008;57: 721–3.
84. de Martel C, Llosa AE, Farr SM, et al. *Helicobacter pylori* infection and the risk of development of esophageal adenocarcinoma. J Infect Dis 2005;191:761–7.
85. Weston AP, Badr AS, Topalovski M, et al. Prospective evaluation of the prevalence of gastric *Helicobacter pylori* infection in patients with GERD, Barrett's esophagus, Barrett's dysplasia, and Barrett's adenocarcinoma. Am J Gastroenterol 2000;95:387–94.
86. Ye W, Held M, Lagergren J, et al. *Helicobacter pylori* infection and gastric atrophy: risk of adenocarcinoma and squamous-cell carcinoma of the esophagus and adenocarcinoma of the gastric cardia. J Natl Cancer Inst 2004;96: 388–96.
87. Anderson LA, Murphy SJ, Johnston BT, et al. Relationship between *Helicobacter pylori* infection and gastric atrophy and the stages of the oesophageal inflammation, metaplasia, adenocarcinoma sequence: results from the FINBAR case-control study. Gut 2008;57:734–9.
88. Chow WH, Blaser MJ, Blot WJ, et al. An inverse relation between *cagA+* strains of *Helicobacter pylori* infection and risk of esophageal and gastric cardia adenocarcinoma. Cancer Res 1998;58:588–90.
89. Rokkas T, Pistiolas D, Sechopoulos P, et al. Relationship between *Helicobacter pylori* infection and esophageal neoplasia: a meta-analysis. Clin Gastroenterol Hepatol 2007;5:1413–7.
90. de Jonge PJ, Steyerberg EW, Kuipers EJ, et al. Risk factors for the development of esophageal adenocarcinoma in Barrett's esophagus. Am J Gastroenterol 2006;101:1421–9.
91. Lindblad M, Rodríguez LA, Lagergren J. Body mass, tobacco and alcohol and risk of esophageal, gastric cardia, and gastric non-cardia adenocarcinoma among men and women in a nested case-control study. Cancer Causes Control 2005;16:285–94.
92. Wu AH, Wan P, Bernstein L. A multiethnic population-based study of smoking, alcohol and body size and risk of adenocarcinomas of the stomach and esophagus (United States). Cancer Causes Control 2001;12:721–32.

93. Vaughan TL, Davis S, Kristal A, et al. Obesity, alcohol, and tobacco as risk factors for cancers of the esophagus and gastric cardia: adenocarcinoma versus squamous cell carcinoma. Cancer Epidemiol Biomarkers Prev 1995;4: 85–92.

94. Gammon MD, Schoenberg JB, Ahsan H, et al. Tobacco, alcohol, and socioeconomic status and adenocarcinomas of the esophagus and gastric cardia. J Natl Cancer Inst 1997;89:1277–84.

95. Brown LM, Silverman DT, Pottern LM, et al. Adenocarcinoma of the esophagus and esophagogastric junction in white men in the United States: alcohol, tobacco, and socioeconomic factors. Cancer Causes Control 1994;5:333–40.

96. Kabat GC, Ng SK, Wynder EL. Tobacco, alcohol intake, and diet in relation to adenocarcinoma of the esophagus and gastric cardia. Cancer Causes Control 1993;4:123–32.

97. Lagergren J, Bergström R, Lindgren A, et al. The role of tobacco, snuff and alcohol use in the aetiology of cancer of the oesophagus and gastric cardia. Int J Cancer 2000;85:340–6.

98. Lagergren J. Adenocarcinoma of oesophagus: what exactly is the size of the problem and who is at risk? Gut 2005;54(Suppl 1):i1–5.

99. Engel LS, Chow WH, Vaughan TL, et al. Population attributable risks of esophageal and gastric cancers. J Natl Cancer Inst 2003;95:1404–13.

100. Navarro Silvera SA, Mayne ST, Risch H, et al. Food group intake and risk of subtypes of esophageal and gastric cancer. Int J Cancer 2008;123:852–60.

101. Chen H, Tucker KL, Graubard BI, et al. Nutrient intakes and adenocarcinoma of the esophagus and distal stomach. Nutr Cancer 2002;42:33–40.

102. Brown LM, Swanson CA, Gridley G, et al. Adenocarcinoma of the esophagus: role of obesity and diet. J Natl Cancer Inst 1995;87:104–9.

103. Thompson CL, Khiani V, Chak A, et al. Carbohydrate consumption and esophageal cancer: an ecological assessment. Am J Gastroenterol 2008;103:555–61.

104. Mayne ST, Risch HA, Dubrow R, et al. Carbonated soft drink consumption and risk of esophageal adenocarcinoma. J Natl Cancer Inst 2006;98:72–5.

105. Lagergren J, Viklund P, Jansson C. Carbonated soft drinks and risk of esophageal adenocarcinoma: a population-based case-control study. J Natl Cancer Inst 2006;98:1158–61.

106. Dong LM, Kristal AR, Peters U, et al. Dietary supplement use and risk of neoplastic progression in esophageal adenocarcinoma: a prospective study. Nutr Cancer 2008;60:39–48.

107. Terry P, Lagergren J, Ye W, et al. Antioxidants and cancers of the esophagus and gastric cardia. Int J Cancer 2000;87:750–4.

108. Corley DA, Kerlikowske K, Verma R, et al. Protective association of aspirin/NSAIDs and esophageal cancer: a systematic review and meta-analysis. Gastroenterology 2003;124:47–56.

109. Funkhouser EM, Sharp GB. Aspirin and reduced risk of esophageal carcinoma. Cancer 1995;76:1116–9.

110. Farrow DC, Vaughan TL, Hansten PD, et al. Use of aspirin and other nonsteroidal anti-inflammatory drugs and risk of esophageal and gastric cancer. Cancer Epidemiol Biomarkers Prev 1998;7:97–102.

111. Vaughan TL, Dong LM, Blount PL, et al. Non-steroidal anti-inflammatory drugs and risk of neoplastic progression in Barrett's oesophagus: a prospective study. Lancet Oncol 2005;6(12):945–52.

112. Jayaprakash V, Menezes RJ, Javle MM, et al. Regular aspirin use and esophageal cancer risk. Int J Cancer 2006;119:202–7.

113. Anderson LA, Johnston BT, Watson RG, et al. Nonsteroidal anti-inflammatory drugs and the esophageal inflammation-metaplasia-adenocarcinoma sequence. Cancer Res 2006;66:4975–82.
114. Lindblad M, Lagergren J, García Rodríguez LA. Nonsteroidal anti-inflammatory drugs and risk of esophageal and gastric cancer. Cancer Epidemiol Biomarkers Prev 2005;14:444–50.
115. Heath EI, Canto MI, Piantadosi S, et al. Chemoprevention for Barrett's Esophagus Trial Research Group. Secondary chemoprevention of Barrett's esophagus with celecoxib: results of a randomized trial. J Natl Cancer Inst 2007;99:545–57.
116. Triadafilopoulos G, Kaur B, Sood S, et al. The effects of esomeprazole combined with aspirin or rofecoxib on prostaglandin E2 production in patients with Barrett's oesophagus. Aliment Pharmacol Ther 2006;23:997–1005.
117. El-Serag HB, Aguirre TV, Davis S, et al. Proton pump inhibitors are associated with reduced incidence of dysplasia in Barrett's esophagus. Am J Gastroenterol 2004;99:1877–83.
118. Hillman LC, Chiragakis L, Shadbolt B, et al. Proton-pump inhibitor therapy and the development of dysplasia in patients with Barrett's oesophagus. Med J Aust 2004;180:387–91.
119. DeMeester S, DeMeester T. Columnar mucosa and intestinal metaplasia of the esophagus: fifty years of controversy. Ann Surg 2000;231:303–21.
120. Ye W, Chow WH, Lagergren J, et al. Risk of adenocarcinomas of the esophagus and gastric cardia in patients with gastroesophageal reflux diseases and after antireflux surgery. Gastroenterology 2001;121:1286–93.
121. Tran T, Spechler SJ, Richardson P, et al. Fundoplication and the risk of esophageal cancer in gastroesophageal reflux disease: a Veterans affairs cohort study. Am J Gastroenterol 2005;100:1002–8.
122. Corey KE, Schmitz SM, Shaheen NJ. Does a surgical antireflux procedure decrease the incidence of esophageal adenocarcinoma in Barrett's esophagus? A meta-analysis. Am J Gastroenterol 2003;98:2390–4.
123. Chang EY, Morris CD, Seltman AK, et al. The effect of antireflux surgery on esophageal carcinogenesis in patients with Barrett esophagus: a systematic review. Ann Surg 2007;246:11–21.
124. Lagergren J, Bergström R, Adami HO, et al. Association between medications that relax the lower esophageal sphincter and risk for esophageal adenocarcinoma. Ann Intern Med 2000;133:165–75.
125. Vaughan TL, Farrow DC, Hansten PD, et al. Risk of esophageal and gastric adenocarcinomas in relation to use of calcium channel blockers, asthma drugs, and other medications that promote gastroesophageal reflux. Cancer Epidemiol Biomarkers Prev 1998;7:749–56.

New Technologies for Imaging of Barrett's Esophagus

Herbert C. Wolfsen, MD[a,b,*]

KEYWORDS

- High resolution endoscopy • Narrow band imaging
- Auto-fluorescence imaging • Confocal endomicroscopy
- Chromoendoscopy • Spectroscopy
- Optical coherence tomography

Several important endoscopic imaging modalities have been recently approved for use and are commercially available. This article reviews these developments and the implications for patients with Barrett's syndrome, especially advanced dysplasia and mucosal carcinoma. The history of Barrett's esophagus has featured important milestones. Norman Barrett's initially described a congenital short esophagus with ulcerations in the gastric cardia. Later, others determined that Barrett's esophagus represented acquired glandular ulcerations of the distal esophagus[1,2] related to severe gastroesophageal reflux disease,[3] with increasing rates of dysplasia and adenocarcinoma.[4] Subsequently, much of the interest in Barrett's esophagus has focused on the utility of standard resolution white light surveillance endoscopy with random mucosal biopsies for the detection of dysplasia and early carcinoma.[5] Recently, important developments in biophotonics have begun to make their way from the laboratory to the gastrointestinal endoscopy unit. Unresolved issues for most of these technologies include regulatory approval, commercial availability, demonstration of clinical utility, securing reimbursement for the required additional time and imaging equipment, and clarifying the medical-legal issues associated with image interpretation and data storage. This article reviews recent developments in endoscopy-based imaging modalities in patients with Barrett's esophagus.

WHITE LIGHT ENDOSCOPIC IMAGING FOR BARRETT'S ESOPHAGUS

Barrett's syndrome is suspected when salmon-colored mucosa in the distal esophagus is detected at endoscopy. North American guidelines require mucosal biopsies

There are no conflicts of interest relating to this publication.

[a] Division of Gastroenterology and Hepatology, Mayo Clinic, 6A Davis Building, 4500 San Pablo Road, Jacksonville, FL 32224, USA

[b] Mayo Medical School, 200 First Street, S.W., Rochester, MN 55905, USA

* Division of Gastroenterology and Hepatology, Mayo Clinic, 6A Davis Building, 4500 San Pablo Road, Jacksonville, FL 32224.

E-mail address: pdt@mayo.edu

to document the specialized intestinal metaplasia of Barrett's syndrome and differentiation from fundic or cardiac forms of gastric metaplasia. Beyond the initial diagnosis, the role of surveillance endoscopy using standard resolution white light surveillance endoscopy has not proven reliable for the visualization of dysplasia and early neoplasia. Therefore, surveillance endoscopy biopsy protocols dependent upon quadrantic mucosal biopsies have been adopted despite their expense, time consumption, associated sampling error, and the high inter- and intraobserver variability found in the histologic analysis.[5,6] Recently, video endoscopes have largely replaced fiberoptic instruments around the world. A video endoscope uses a charge-coupled device (CCD)—an integrated electrical circuit made of photosensitive silicone semiconductors. The CCD surface is made up of photosensitive elements (pixels) that generate an electrical charge in proportion to light exposure and then generate an analog signal that is digitalized by the computer video processor. CCDs in standard video endoscopes have 100,000 to 300,000 pixels and the image resolution, the ability to discriminate between two adjacent points, varies accordingly. These endoscopes have a focal distance of 1 to 9 cm and images will appear out of focus if they are beyond this range. Endoscopes with high-density CCDs (600,000–1,000,000 pixels per CCD) are referred to as high-resolution endoscopes (HRE). They are capable of producing high-magnification images with increased spatial resolution for the detection of minute abnormalities in mucosal glandular and vascular structures. In conjunction with a movable lens for magnification endoscopy, the focal distance may be controlled to allow detailed examination of the mucosal surface at close range (<3 mm).

CHROMOENDOSCOPY FOR BARRETT'S ESOPHAGUS

The use of HRE with high-magnification endoscopy over a large mucosal surface area is laborious and impractical. Therefore, HRE and magnification endoscopy have been combined with chromoendoscopy (vital dye staining with agents such as Lugol iodine solution, methylene blue, indigo carmine, crystal violet, and acetic acid) in an attempt to improve detection of mucosal abnormalities. The use of chromoendoscopy for the enhanced detection of the specialized intestinal metaplasia of Barrett's esophagus has been recently reviewed.[7] Lugol solution (a 0.5%–3.0% aqueous solution of potassium iodide and iodine) is used to improve the detection and delineation of the squamous cell carcinoma and dysplasia in the aerodigestive tract by way of absorption by glycogen-containing cells. Lugol is often used with endoscopy procedures in patients at increased risk of squamous cell carcinoma (heavy smokers, alcoholics, and prior lye-ingestion patients). Methylene blue (0.1%–1.0% solution after mucolysis) is used for detection of Barrett's esophagus as it is taken up by intestinalized mucosa but not squamous or gastric mucosa. Methylene blue, indigo carmine, and acetic acid combined with magnification endoscopy have been found to identify mucosal glandular patterns. Guelrud and colleagues[8] described four pit patterns using acetic acid and magnification endoscopy (round, reticular, villous, and ridged), and found ridged and villous to be associated with intestinal metaplasia. Sharma and colleagues[9] described three mucosal patterns visualized with indigo carmine in patients with Barrett's esophagus (ridged-villous, circular, irregular-distorted) with the ridged or villous patterns found be associated with intestinal metaplasia, while the irregular or distorted pattern was noted with Barrett's high-grade dysplasia (HGD) or superficial adenocarcinoma. A review of seven prospective and controlled studies using methylene blue-targeted biopsies found a higher yield for the detection of Barrett's syndrome compared with a random biopsy protocol.[8,10–15] Sharma and colleagues[9] studied 80 Barrett's esophagus patients using indigo carmine dye and determined the presence of the ridged or villous pattern had high sensitivity, specificity, and positive predictive value (97%, 76%, and 92%, respectively). The distorted or irregular glandular pattern was also detected in six patients with Barrett's HGD. However, subsequent studies have failed to demonstrate a detection benefit for either Barrett's metaplasia or dysplasia.[16,17] There was also a report that raises the issue of DNA damage resulting from methylene blue staining and white light illumination.[18] Similar conflicting results have been found with studies using acetic acid (a mucolytic agent that alters cellular protein structure) and crystal violet staining.[19–21] These initial enthusiastic results have subsequently been found to vary widely, perhaps related to differences in technique, operator experience, and patient population with the prevalence of Barrett's esophagus.[7,22] A study among four expert gastrointestinal endoscopists in Europe analyzed blinded evaluations of magnification chromoendoscopy images of Barrett's esophagus using acetic acid or methylene blue. The interobserver agreement was poor (kappa = 0.40) for all parameters studied—including the mucosal patterns, methylene blue positive staining, and the presence of specialized intestinal metaplasia. These inconsistencies, along with safety issues, and increased cost and procedure time, have prevented the widespread use of vital dye staining chromoendoscopy techniques.[23]

NARROW-BAND IMAGING FOR BARRETT'S ESOPHAGUS

Narrow-band imaging (NBI) is currently the best-studied, advanced endoscopic-imaging technique for the detection of Barrett's dysplasia. NBI has received regulatory approval and is a commercially available method of optical chromoendoscopy that improves detection of mucosal abnormalities without the messy, time-consuming problems associated with vital dye staining chromoendoscopy. NBI was developed by Gono and colleagues[24] in 1999 as a joint project of the Japanese National Cancer Center Hospital East and Olympus Corporation (Tokyo, Japan). Their team of bio-optical physicists studied variations of conventional endoscopy that potentially could visualize early changes of angiogenesis (increased density of microvessels) associated with the development of dysplasia and superficial neoplasia. Using light filters, the contribution of blue light is increased by narrowing the band widths of the red, green, and blue components of the excitation light; reducing the amount of green light; and eliminating the red light. The resulting "narrow band" blue-green light improves imaging of mucosal patterns because of the limited optical scattering and shallow penetration depth. This blue light is also absorbed by hemoglobin (since the hemoglobin absorption band—Soret band—lies at 415 nm) for optimal detection of mucosal glandular and vascular patterns, and the presence of abnormal blood vessels that are associated with the development of dysplasia.[25]

Several single-center studies have correlated the appearance of mucosal glandular and vascular patterns with metaplasia. Kara and colleagues[26] studied magnified images in Barrett's esophagus patients and found that regular mucosal and vascular patterns were associated intestinal metaplasia; whereas irregular mucosal and vascular patterns and the presence of abnormal blood vessels were associated with Barrett's HGD. These mucosal and vascular patterns have been the basis of a series of studies (from several advanced-endoscopy centers) that have demonstrated the utility of NBI in evaluating Barrett's dysplasia patients. Kara and colleagues compared HRE with indigo carmine chromoendoscopy or NBI in 14 patients with Barrett's HGD. The aim of the study was to test and compare these combinations for the detection of Barrett's HGD or superficial carcinoma. HRE alone found HGD in 11 patients (79%), NBI detected 12 patients (86%), and indigo carmine chromoendoscopy detected 13 patients (93%). One patient had HGD that was not detected with any imaging modality and found only with random biopsies (7%). NBI found an additional four HGD lesions in 3 of these 12 patients. The efficacy of the techniques was found to be similar. NBI was preferred over vital dye staining for its ease of use. White light HRE detected all cases of HGD, suggesting that NBI should be used for detailed inspection of suspicious lesions, rather than for their primary detection. As a historical analysis, these findings were compared with previous studies using standard resolution white light endoscopy in Barrett's esophagus where HGD was detected using targeted biopsies in 62% of patients. However, using targeted biopsies plus random four quadrant biopsies found HGD in 85% of patients. Although not directly compared, the use of NBI seems to be as good, or better, than the use of standard resolution endoscopy (SRE)-targeted plus random biopsies.[27–29] Anagnostopoulos and colleagues[27] found similar results in a study of 344 lesions in 50 patients using magnified endoscopic microstructural and vascular features of Barrett's syndrome. Regular microstructural patterns associated with sensitivity, specificity, and positive and negative predictive values of 100%, 79%, 94%, and 100%, respectively for the detection of intestinal metaplasia. The sensitivity, specificity, and positive and negative predictive values for the detection of HGD was 90%, 100%, 99%, and 100%, respectively.[27] A recent article from Curvers and colleagues[30] studied the use of HRE with vital dye staining techniques using acetic acid, indigo carmine, and NBI in 14 patients with 22 suspicious lesions (8 areas of HGD, 1 area of low-grade dysplasia [LGD], 1 area indefinite for dysplasia, and 12 areas of nondysplastic Barrett's syndrome). Seven community and five expert gastrointestinal endoscopists evaluated standard images from these lesions, in a blinded manner, to evaluate the glandular and vascular patterns and association with dysplasia. The yield for detecting dysplasia or neoplasia with white light HRE was 86% overall (90% for experts and 84% for nonexperts) and the addition of enhancement techniques (vital dye staining or NBI) did not improve the diagnostic yield.[30]

A prospective, blinded, tandem endoscopy study from the author's group,[31] compared SRE and HRE-NBI in 65 patients referred for evaluation of Barrett's dysplasia. As commercially available HRE-NBI systems in North America do not have high-magnification capability, the determination of areas suspicious for dysplasia or cancer was made with standard endoscopic techniques in an attempt to reproduce a realistic clinical practice setting. This study found that NBI-targeted biopsies found dysplasia in more patients (37 patients, 57%) compared with SRE-targeted plus random biopsies (28 patients, 43%; $P<.001$). NBI also found higher grades of dysplasia in 12 patients (18%) compared with no patients in whom SRE-targeted and random biopsies detected a high grade of histology (0%; $P<.001$). In addition, more biopsies were taken using SRE- targeted plus random biopsies (mean 8.5 biopsies per case) compared with NBI-directed biopsies (mean 4.7 biopsies per case; $P<.001$). The ability of HRE combined with NBI to find dysplasia in significantly more patients with Barrett's esophagus with greater efficiency (using significantly fewer biopsy samples) illustrates the importance of this technology for the surveillance evaluation of Barrett's esophagus patients. Further studies will be required to document this increased efficiency and cost savings for surveillance endoscopy and to determine the impact of HRE-NBI on the results of endoscopic screening and surveillance programs for dysplasia detection in Barrett's esophagus.[32,33]

AUTOFLUORESCENCE IMAGING FOR BARRETT'S ESOPHAGUS

Autofluorescence imaging (AFI) is a technique that differentiates tissue types based on their differences in fluorescence emission. When tissues are exposed to short- wavelength light, endogenous biologic substances (fluorophores) are excited causing emission of fluorescent light of a longer wavelength (autofluorescence). The molecules responsible for tissue autofluorescence include collagen, NADH, elastin, flavin, porphyrins, and aromatic amino acids—each with a characteristic excitation and emission spectral pattern. AFI detects differences in the natural, endogenous fluorescence of normal, dysplastic, and neoplastic mucosa using blue light illumination producing a low-intensity autofluorescence that is detected through highly sensitive CCDs, along with reflectance imaging detected through a nonintensified CCD.[34] The image processor incorporates the CCD signals into a real-time pseudocolor image of normal mucosa (green color) and dysplasia or neoplasia (varying tones of red or purple color). Previously, AFI was used with fiberoptic endoscopes that provided relatively poor white light images. Representative examples of comparative Barrett's HGD viewed with high-resolution white light, narrow band, and AFIs are demonstrated in **Figs. 1** through **6**. Early studies with this limited technology proved no benefit for the use of AFI over white light endoscopy—including a randomized, crossover study from the Academic Medical Center in Amsterdam.[29,35,36] In a single-center, uncontrolled study, Kara and colleagues evaluated the use of AFI after white light HRE in 60 patients with Barrett's esophagus. HGD was detected in 22 patients, including 6 patients where no lesion was identified with white light endoscopy and found only with AFI. Therefore, AFI detected a significant number of patients with HGD who had no visible lesions on white light HRE, increasing the target detection rate from 63% to 91%. However, the use of AFI was associated with a 51% false-positive rate since 41 of 81 suspicious areas detected by AFI did not have dysplasia at biopsy. AFI endoscopy, then, offers the promise of wide-area imaging for Barrett's surveillance, but is associated with poor specificity.[37]

Subsequently, trimodal imaging endoscopes have been developed that combine the use of widefield endoscopic imaging (white light HRE), a widefield sensitive method for the detection of dysplasia and carcinoma (so-called "red flag" technique; AFI), and a virtual chromoendoscopy technique (NBI). This enhances and improves the combined accuracy of these techniques for the detection of mucosal dysplasia and neoplasia (NBI).[38] Again, the initial single-center study was from Amsterdam, where 20 patients were evaluated for 47 suspicious areas found with AFI. Of these 47 areas, 28 were found to be abnormal based on NBI. Subsequently, biopsy confirmed the diagnosis of HGD in each case. However, 14 of 19 areas detected with AFI appeared normal with NBI, thereby reducing the number of false-positive lesions from 40% to

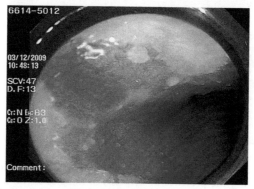

Fig. 1. Peninsula of glandular epithelium at proximal margin of long segment Barrett's esophagus, viewed with high-resolution white light.

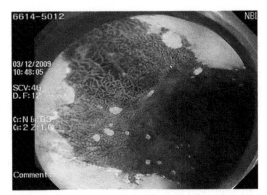

Fig. 2. NBI demonstrating enhanced glandular and vascular abnormalities of focal HGD, biopsy proven. Reviewing **Fig. 1**, the NBI-detected area of dysplasia is more easily identified as an area of deeper red color with surface granularity. This phenomenon has been described as the ability of NBI to improve Barrett's dysplasia detection using only white light endoscopy.

10% (of 47 lesions, total). With HGD, the positive predictive value of AFI alone for Barrett's syndrome was only 60%, but improved to 85% in combination with NBI.[39] Curvers and colleagues[31] have just published the results of using trimodal imaging in four expert endoscopy-imaging centers in Europe and the United States for the evaluation of 84 patients referred with Barrett's dysplasia. The study outcomes used were the number of patients and lesions of HGD detected with HRE and AFI, plus the reduction of false-positive AFI findings after NBI. The AFI algorithm used total autofluorescence after blue light illumination and green reflectance. At endoscopy, HRE was first used to examine the Barrett's segment for the presence of esophagitis or visible lesions. Then, AFI was used to identify areas suspicious for the presence of dysplasia (violet-purple pseudocolor). NBI was then used to describe the vascular and mucosal pattern of these suspicious lesions to determine if they were suspicious for the presence of dysplasia. Random quadrantic biopsies were obtained after the image-targeted biopsies.

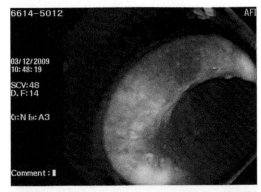

Fig. 3. Trimodal image (XGIF-Q260FZ, Olympus Inc., Tokyo, Japan) with corresponding AFI demonstrating the dark purple mucosal pseudocolor based on the pattern of endogenous fluorescence, suggesting the presence of dysplasia or neoplasia. The surrounding mucosa appears green in the AFI pseudocolor image indicating normal fluorescence patterns (no dysplasia).

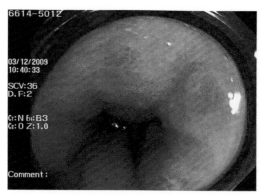

Fig. 4. Nodule of raised, hyperemic mucosa at the 2:00 location found within a long-segment Barrett's esophagus, viewed with high-resolution white light.

Overall, 30 patients were diagnosed with Barrett's HGD. Sixteen cases were detected with HRE, 11 were detected only with AFI, and 3 were diagnosed only by random biopsies. The use of AFI, therefore, increased the number of patients found to have HGD from 53% (16 of 30 patients) to 90% (27 of 30 patients). The use of NBI reduced the false-positive rate of AFI from 81% to 26% and the false-positive rate of HRE from 67% to 44%, but misclassified two lesions that were found to contain HGD. The utility of random quadrantic biopsies in addition to HRE, AFI, and NBI is unknown. Thus far, the published experience with these prototype systems combining the use of HRE, AFI, and NBI in one endoscope has come from academic centers with expert endoscopists who evaluate a highly selected group of Barrett's patients with dysplasia and carcinoma. The application of this technology has not yet been studied in other practice settings and these devices have not been approved for use in the United States.

CONFOCAL FLUORESCENCE MICROSCOPY FOR BARRETT'S ESOPHAGUS

The development of probe-based and endoscopic devices for real-time, in vivo microscopic imaging of Barrett's mucosa represents another milestone in advanced imaging technology.[40] Confocal microscopy uses stimulation mucosal cells with

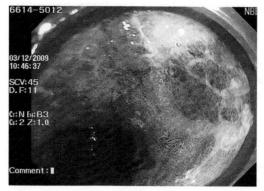

Fig. 5. NBI identifying the nodule clearly. Note the diffuse glandular and vascular abnormalities of focal HGD found throughout most of this field of Barrett's esophagus, especially in the 9:00 to 12:00 quadrant.

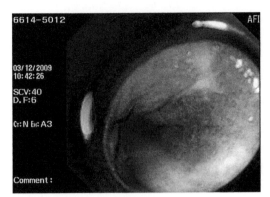

Fig. 6. Trimodal image (XGIF-Q260FZ, Olympus Inc., Tokyo, Japan) with corresponding AFI demonstrating the dark purple pseudocolor throughout this field of Barrett's syndrome indicating extensive HGD. The AFI green-appearing mucosa in the lower quadrants indicates normal fluorescence patterns (no dysplasia).

blue laser light that is reflected back through a pinhole opening to eliminate out-of-focus light. Laser scanning with computer-generated, cross-sectional images permits real-time microscopic imaging of Barrett's mucosa. The miniature confocal microscope developed by OptiScan (Pentax, Japan), permits magnification beyond ×1,000 with cellular and subcellular resolution of crypt and cellular architecture to a depth of 250 microns (level of the lamina propria). Improved images require the use of a contrast agent such as topical acriflavine or intravenous fluorescein sodium for resolution of cellular structures and microvasculature. Image production tends to be relatively slow (one frame per second), creating lengthy procedure times. Initial studies using this system have reported very high accuracy (85%–94%) for the detection of HGD in Barrett's esophagus.[41,42] However, these results reflect the expert use of this technology in a single referral center. This microscopy analysis was performed in patients with visible lesions detected on white light endoscopy. It is unclear if this experience would produce similar results for lesions that were not visible with white light endoscopy or if this technology could produce similar or significantly better results when compared with trimodal imaging with HRE, AFI, and NBI.

The second approach to in vivo microscopic imaging involves a small confocal microscope probe developed by Mauna Kea Technologies, France, which can be used with any endoscope to provide real-time endoscopic microscopy to varying depths from 50 to 200 microns.[43] This system features postprocedure image reconstruction for video mosaicing—the combination of dynamic single frame images into a static, mosaic image over a broad field without reduction in image resolution.[44] Larger studies from more centers are needed to determine the role and utility of confocal microendoscopy systems in the evaluation of patients with Barrett's syndrome.

ENDOCYTOSCOPY FOR BARRETT'S ESOPHAGUS

Endocytoscopy allows visualization of cells and nuclei using high-magnification probes or endoscopes for the detection of dysplasia, neoplasia, inflammation, and infection involving the gut mucosa with initial reports describing findings in 12 esophageal squamous cell cancer patients.[45] For use in Barrett's syndrome, this method requires a dye or contrast agent such as methylene blue or NBI for cellular imaging to evaluate the cell size, shape, and nuclear characteristics. A recent ex vivo study of 166 biopsy sites from 16 patients with ×450 and ×1125 magnification while blinded to endoscopic and histologic findings found adenocarcinoma in 4.2% of biopsy sites, high-grade intraepithelial neoplasia in 16.9%, and low-grade intraepithelial neoplasia in 12.1%. Adequate assessment of endocytoscopy images was not possible in 49% of the target areas at the ×450 magnification and in 22% of the target areas at ×1125 magnification. At most, 23% of images with lower magnification and 41% of higher magnification images could be interpreted to identify characteristics of dysplasia and neoplasia. Interobserver agreement was less than fair (kappa from <0 to 0.45) with positive and negative predictive values for HGD or carcinoma of 0.29 and 0.87, respectively, for ×450 magnification and 0.44 and 0.83, respectively, for ×1125 magnification.[46] The real-time, in vivo use of these systems is likely to be limited by image stabilization problems with motion artifact and image distortion.

SPECTROSCOPY FOR BARRETT'S ESOPHAGUS

Optical spectroscopy may provide the means to detect mucosal abnormalities in real time using molecular and microstructural information in light-tissue interactions such as fluorescence, reflectance (elastic scattering), and Raman (inelastic scattering).[47] The behavior of light provides information about tissue composition, oxygenation, degree of inflammation, and dysplasia for histologic-like characterizations of gut mucosa. Different spectroscopic techniques can be used to provide information about tissue biochemistry and oxygenation. Currently available clinical studies are limited to single-center feasibility studies. Reflectance spectroscopy quantitatively measures the color and intensity of reflected light after tissue illumination to discriminate normal, dysplastic, and neoplastic mucosa. Unlike autofluorescence spectroscopy, this reflected light maintains the same wavelength, although varying degrees of light wavelengths are absorbed and reflected. Hemoglobin is the primary molecule that absorbs light, providing a marker of angiogenesis and dysplasia based on tissue oxygenation. Light-scattering spectroscopy (LSS) is a type of reflectance spectroscopy that studies elastic scattering (light not changed by the tissue interaction). Each wavelength of light is scattered differently depending on the density of the mucosal and cellular structures it encounters. By measuring which light wavelengths are scattered, and which are not, the size and characteristics of the mucosal and cellular structures may be determined. Since endogenous fluorophores produce weak fluorescence signals, exogenous fluorophores such as porphyrin compounds are used to enhance the fluorescence effect. Exogenous fluorophores seem to be specifically retained in dysplastic and neoplastic tissue, and exhibit an induced fluorescence signal of much higher intensity. Among different sensitizers, porphyrins have been the most studied for application in fluorescence spectroscopy. Porphyrins are heme products that are associated with prolonged photosensitivity (porfimer sodium) or other potentially serious adverse events such as nausea and hypotension (amino levulinic acid). The advantage of drug-induced fluorescence is that the fluorescent signal generated by these exogenous fluorophores is typically stronger than autofluorescence and can be detected by simpler and cheaper instruments. Among exogenous fluorophores, 5-aminolevulinic acid (5-ALA) is the most studied photosensitizer that is converted intracellularly to the photoactive compound protoporphyrin IX, which is associated with a significantly higher tumor selectivity compared with other exogenous fluorophores used in fluorescence imaging.[48] Furthermore, compared with other exogenous fluorophores, skin sensitivity is reduced to 24 to 48 hours although cardiovascular side effects, including severe hypotension and sudden death, have been reported.[49,50] An issue in the measurement of fluorescence spectra is the background generated by scattering and absorption. In this case, the fluorescence spectra may be analyzed with information from the corresponding reflectance spectra to permit subtraction of this background and produce a measure of intrinsic fluorescence.[51] Different fluorophores are excited by different wavelengths of light and the optimal excitation wavelength for detecting dysplasia is unknown. A significant technical advance in fluorescence spectroscopy was made with the development of a fast multiexcitation system capable of rapid tissue excitation with up to 11 wavelengths that provide information to optical probes allowing collection of many different fluorescence spectra for the determination of the optimal excitation wavelength.[51,52] In addition to specific excitation and emission wavelengths, different fluorophores fade or decay their fluorescence at varying rates. This difference between normal and abnormal tissue can be enhanced by measuring stimulated fluorescence at different intervals. This technique, termed "time-resolved fluorescence," has been used to increase the accuracy of dysplasia detection in patients with Barrett's esophagus.[53]

Light propagation in tissue is governed by scattering and absorption. LSS measures the extent to which the angular path of photons of light is altered by the size and number of cellular components (scatterers) they encounter. The primary scatterers are collagen fibers in the extracellular matrix, mitochondria, cellular nuclei, and other intracellular structures. By mathematical modeling, the number, size, and optical density of cellular structures (such as nuclei), can be determined by measuring the diffuse reflected light from epithelial surfaces.[54] This phenomenon has been exploited during endoscopic procedures to determine the number of nuclei, the size of nuclei, and the degree of crowding of nuclei in patients with dysplastic changes in Barrett's esophagus.[55,56] These studies have demonstrated that light scattering can accurately determine nuclear size, detect abnormally enlarged nuclei, and characterize different grades of dysplasia with less interobserver variability than routine pathology. Unlike fluorescence, LSS uses a broad range of light to detect changes over the entire visible spectrum. Reflectance spectroscopy, laser-induced autofluorescence spectroscopy, and LSS provide quantitative information that characterize either biochemical or morphologic aspects of tissue that can be significantly altered during the development of neoplasia. This improves the distinction of dysplastic and normal tissue by combining the information provided by each of the spectroscopic techniques obtained simultaneously with trimodal spectroscopy.

Raman spectroscopy detects scattered light that has been slightly shifted in wavelength (inelastic scattering) resulting from energy transfer between light and mucosa molecules. These shifts correspond to specific vibrations of molecular bonds. Since some of the light energy is transferred to the molecule in this process, the light emitted back from the tissue is reduced in energy and has a longer wavelength. Raman spectra consist of multiple peaks and bands that may produce detailed tissue characterization. However, this Raman signal is very weak and near infrared light is typically used for excitation; and sophisticated detection instruments and signal processing computers are required. Raman spectroscopy has recently been applied to the detection of Barrett's-associated dysplasia with promising results.[57,58]

Panjehpour and colleagues[59] studied laser-induced autofluorescence using a wavelength of 410 nm to distinguish normal esophageal mucosa from dysplastic and malignant tissue with high accuracy. Using a different spectral analysis technique, Vo-Dinh and colleagues[60] were also able to detect esophageal carcinoma with a high degree of reliability. The same group of investigators found laser-induced autofluorescence spectroscopy to be sensitive for the detection of diffuse HGD in Barrett's esophagus and adenocarcinoma. However, only 28% of the specimens with LGD and focal HGD were classified as abnormal by this technique.[61] Mayinger and colleagues[62] used a filtered ultraviolet-blue light source and showed specific differences in the emitted autofluorescence spectra of esophageal carcinoma with normal mucosa. Bourg-Heckly and colleagues[63] demonstrated the ability of light-induced autofluorescence to identify HGD in Barrett's esophagus and early cancer, and reported a sensitivity and specificity of 86% and 95%, respectively. Curiously, this technique could not distinguish nondysplastic Barrett's mucosa from squamous mucosa. Some investigators used exogenous fluorophores to enhance the spectroscopic characteristics of dysplastic and neoplastic tissues. von Holstein and colleagues[64] demonstrated the feasibility of laser-induced fluorescence measurements using the photosensitizer porfimer sodium (Photofrin; Axcan, Mont St Hilaire, Quebec, Canada) to distinguish normal and malignant tissue in an in vitro study of esophagectomy specimens. Brand and colleagues[65] performed a similar study using the oral photosensitizer 5-ALA that found a sensitivity of 77% and specificity of 71%. Ortner and colleagues[53] combined time-resolved fluorescence spectroscopy and topical application of 5-ALA to enhance the spectroscopic characteristics of dysplastic Barrett's esophagus. LSS and trimodal spectroscopy are novel techniques and few data are available. Perelman and colleagues[54] described the use of LSS to determine the size distribution of epithelial cell nuclei in vitro and in vivo; and Wallace and colleagues[55,56] reported a prospective validation study of LSS to identify dysplasia in a cohort of patients with Barrett's esophagus. The sensitivity and specificity of LSS for detecting dysplasia (either LGD or HGD) were each 90%; with all HGD and 87% of LGD sites correctly classified. In a tandem study, Georgakoudi and colleagues[51] found the combination of laser-induced autofluorescence, reflectance, and LSS (used together, referred to as trimodal spectroscopy) resulted in improved sensitivity and specificity for the distinction of HGD versus non–high-grade dysplasia in Barrett's esophagus (each 100%); and dysplastic versus non-dysplastic Barrett's esophagus (93% and 100%, respectively). Despite the relatively promising results reported in many of these feasibility studies, continued improvement in these detection and signal-processing devices will be required to justify the time and expense associated with the large clinical trials that will ultimately be required for assessment, validation, regulatory approval, and commercial production.

OPTICAL COHERENCE TOMOGRAPHY FOR BARRETT'S ESOPHAGUS

Optical coherence tomography (OCT) uses short coherence-length, broadband light for micrometer-sized, cross-sectional imaging of the gut mucosa that is similar to endoscopic ultrasound—except that it uses light instead of sound.[66] First used in 1997, time domain OCT systems had limited image speed, and sensitivity.[67] Recently, the development of Fourier domain OCT has provided much greater imaging speed, sensitivity, and potential to perform three dimensional imaging in real-time. The limited development of the image detection devices (scanning probes) has made clinical application cumbersome and impractical, thus far.[68,69]

CONCLUSIONS AND THE FUTURE OF IMAGING FOR BARRETT'S ESOPHAGUS

Some of endoscopy-based imaging technologies for the detection of Barrett's syndrome, dysplasia, and neoplasia in patients with Barrett's esophagus have already achieved regulatory approval, commercial availability, and establishment of clinical utility and practical application (albeit in academic referral endoscopy centers). Important examples include white light HRE and NBI. Validation studies are ongoing for use of the endoscopic trimodal imaging system that combines widefield detection capabilities of HRE and AFI with improved sensitivity (and reduced numbers of false-positive results) with NBI. Regulatory approval for the use of the combination systems has already been granted in Europe and approval in the United States is expected soon.

The use of endomicroscopy and spectroscopy techniques, especially endoscopic laser confocal microscopy, are being aggressively studied as the most clinically advanced spectroscopic method of "optical biopsy" currently available in commercial systems. The future of imaging for Barrett's syndrome likely rests with the development of molecular targeting with dysplasia-targeted probes (such as monoclonal antibodies) that have been conjugated to dyes or nanoparticles (such as quantum dots or Q dots). These sensitive and specific devices will serve as diagnostic molecular beacons and as a delivery system for therapeutic agents.[47] Several important issues are unresolved, including regulatory approval, demonstration of clinical utility, securing additional reimbursement for the required procedure time and imaging equipment, and clarifying the medical and liability issues associated with the interpretation and storage of these images.

REFERENCES

1. Allison PR. Peptic ulcer of the esophagus. Thorax 1948;3(0):20–42.
2. Allison PR, Johnstone AS. The oesophagus lined with gastric mucous membrane. Thorax 1953;8(2):87–101.
3. Iascone C, DeMeester TR, Little AG, et al. Barrett's esophagus. Functional assessment, proposed pathogenesis, and surgical therapy. Arch Surg 1983;118(5):543–9.
4. Blot WJ, Devesa SS, Kneller RW, et al. Rising incidence of adenocarcinoma of the esophagus and gastric cardia. JAMA 1991;265(10):1287–9.
5. Provenzale D, Kemp JA, Arora S, et al. A guide for surveillance of patients with Barrett's esophagus. Am J Gastroenterol 1994;89(5):670–80.
6. Schlemper RJ, Riddell RH, Kato Y, et al. The Vienna classification of gastrointestinal epithelial neoplasia. Gut 2000;47(2):251–5.
7. Canto MI. Chromoendoscopy and magnifying endoscopy for Barrett's esophagus. Clin Gastroenterol Hepatol 2005;3(7 Suppl 1):S12–5.
8. Guelrud M, Herrera I, Essenfeld H, et al. Enhanced magnification endoscopy: a new technique to identify specialized intestinal metaplasia in Barrett's esophagus. Gastrointest Endosc 2001;53(6):559–65.
9. Sharma P, Weston AP, Topalovski M, et al. Magnification chromoendoscopy for the detection of intestinal metaplasia and dysplasia in Barrett's oesophagus. Gut 2003;52(1):24–7.
10. Fortun PJ, Anagnostopoulos GK, Kaye P, et al. Acetic acid-enhanced magnification endoscopy in the diagnosis of specialized intestinal metaplasia, dysplasia and early cancer in Barrett's oesophagus. Aliment Pharmacol Ther 2006;23(6):735–42.
11. Hamamoto Y, Endo T, Nosho K, et al. Usefulness of narrow-band imaging endoscopy for diagnosis of Barrett's esophagus. J Gastroenterol 2004;39(1):14–20.
12. Kouklakis GS, Kountouras J, Dokas SM, et al. Methylene blue chromoendoscopy for the detection of Barrett's esophagus in a Greek cohort. Endoscopy 2003; 35(5):383–7.
13. Canto MI, Setrakian S, Willis JE, et al. Methylene blue staining of dysplastic and nondysplastic Barrett's esophagus: an in vivo and ex vivo study. Endoscopy 2001;33(5):391–400.
14. Canto MI, Setrakian S, Willis J, et al. Methylene blue-directed biopsies improve detection of intestinal metaplasia and dysplasia in Barrett's esophagus. Gastrointest Endosc 2000;51(5):560–8.

15. Sharma P, Topalovski M, Mayo MS, et al. Methylene blue chromoendoscopy for detection of short-segment Barrett's esophagus. Gastrointest Endosc 2001; 54(3):289–93.
16. Wo JM, Ray MB, Mayfield-Stokes S, et al. Comparison of methylene blue-directed biopsies and conventional biopsies in the detection of intestinal metaplasia and dysplasia in Barrett's esophagus: a preliminary study. Gastrointest Endosc 2001;54(3):294–301.
17. Lim CH, Rotimi O, Dexter SP, et al. Randomized crossover study that used methylene blue or random 4-quadrant biopsy for the diagnosis of dysplasia in Barrett's esophagus. Gastrointest Endosc 2006;64(2):195–9.
18. Olliver JR, Wild CP, Sahay P, et al. Chromoendoscopy with methylene blue and associated DNA damage in Barrett's oesophagus. Lancet 2003;362(9381):373–4.
19. Ferguson DD, DeVault KR, Krishna M, et al. Enhanced magnification-directed biopsies do not increase the detection of intestinal metaplasia in patients with GERD. Am J Gastroenterol 2006;101(7):1611–6.
20. Amano Y, Kushiyama Y, Ishihara S, et al. Crystal violet chromoendoscopy with mucosal pit pattern diagnosis is useful for surveillance of short-segment Barrett's esophagus. Am J Gastroenterol 2005;100(1):21–6.
21. Hoffman A, Kiesslich R, Bender A, et al. Acetic acid-guided biopsies after magnifying endoscopy compared with random biopsies in the detection of Barrett's esophagus: a prospective randomized trial with crossover design. Gastrointest Endosc 2006;64(1):1–8.
22. Armstrong D. Review article: towards consistency in the endoscopic diagnosis of Barrett's oesophagus and columnar metaplasia. Aliment Pharmacol Ther 2004; 20(Suppl 5):40–7, discussion 61–2.
23. Canto MI, Kalloo A. Chromoendoscopy for Barrett's esophagus in the twenty-first century: to stain or not to stain? Gastrointest Endosc 2006;64(2):200–5.
24. Gono K, Obi T, Yamaguchi M, et al. Appearance of enhanced tissue features in narrow-band endoscopic imaging. J Biomed Opt 2004;9(3):568–77.
25. Sharma P, Bansal A, Mathur S, et al. The utility of a novel narrow band imaging endoscopy system in patients with Barrett's esophagus. Gastrointest Endosc 2006;64(2):167–75.
26. Kara MA, Ennahachi M, Fockens P, et al. Detection and classification of the mucosal and vascular patterns (mucosal morphology) in Barrett's esophagus by using narrow band imaging. Gastrointest Endosc 2006;64(2):155–66.
27. Anagnostopoulos GK, Yao K, Kaye P, et al. Novel endoscopic observation in Barrett's oesophagus using high resolution magnification endoscopy and narrow band imaging. Aliment Pharmacol Ther 2007;26(3):501–7.
28. Kara MA, Smits ME, Rosmolen WD, et al. A randomized crossover study comparing light-induced fluorescence endoscopy with standard videoendoscopy for the detection of early neoplasia in Barrett's esophagus. Gastrointest Endosc 2005;61(6):671–8.
29. Kara MA, Peters FP, Rosmolen WD, et al. High-resolution endoscopy plus chromoendoscopy or narrow-band imaging in Barrett's esophagus: a prospective randomized crossover study. Endoscopy 2005;37(10):929–36.
30. Curvers WL, Singh R, Wong Kee Song LM, et al. Endoscopic tri-modal imaging for detection of early neoplasia in Barrett's oesophagus; A multi-centre feasibility study using high-resolution endoscopy, autofluorescence imaging and narrow band imaging incorporated in one endoscopy system. Gut 2008;57:167–72.
31. Wolfsen HC, Crook JE, Krishna M, et al. Prospective, controlled tandem endoscopy study of narrow band imaging for dysplasia detection in Barrett's esophagus. Gastroenterology 2008;135(1):24–31.

32. Sharma P, Bansal A. Toward better imaging of Barrett's esophagus—see more, biopsy less!. Gastrointest Endosc 2006;64(2):188–92.

33. Gheorghe C. Narrow-band imaging endoscopy for diagnosis of malignant and premalignant gastrointestinal lesions. J Gastrointestin Liver Dis 2006;15(1): 77–82.

34. Kara M, DaCosta RS, Wilson BC, et al. Autofluorescence-based detection of early neoplasia in patients with Barrett's esophagus. Dig Dis 2004;22(2):134–41.

35. Niepsuj K, Niepsuj G, Cebula W, et al. Autofluorescence endoscopy for detection of high-grade dysplasia in short-segment Barrett's esophagus. Gastrointest Endosc 2003;58(5):715–9.

36. Egger K, Werner M, Meining A, et al. Biopsy surveillance is still necessary in patients with Barrett's oesophagus despite new endoscopic imaging techniques. Gut 2003;52(1):18–23.

37. Kara MA, Peters FP, Ten Kate FJ, et al. Endoscopic video autofluorescence imaging may improve the detection of early neoplasia in patients with Barrett's esophagus. Gastrointest Endosc 2005;61(6):679–85.

38. Mackenzie G, Lovat L. Advances in diagnostic endoscopy. Medicine 2007;35(6): 330–2.

39. Kara MA, Peters FP, Fockens P, et al. Endoscopic video-autofluorescence imaging followed by narrow band imaging for detecting early neoplasia in Barrett's esophagus. Gastrointest Endosc 2006;64(2):176–85.

40. Kiesslich R, Burg J, Vieth M, et al. Confocal laser endoscopy for diagnosing intra-epithelial neoplasias and colorectal cancer in vivo. Gastroenterology 2004; 127(3):706–13.

41. Polglase AL, McLaren WJ, Skinner SA, et al. A fluorescence confocal endomicro-scope for in vivo microscopy of the upper- and the lower-GI tract. Gastrointest Endosc 2005;62(5):686–95.

42. Kiesslich R, Gossner L, Goetz M, et al. In vivo histology of Barrett's esophagus and associated neoplasia by confocal laser endomicroscopy. Clin Gastroenterol Hepatol 2006;4(8):979–87.

43. Meining A, Saur D, Bajbouj M, et al. In vivo histopathology for detection of gastro-intestinal neoplasia with a portable, confocal miniprobe: an examiner blinded analysis. Clin Gastroenterol Hepatol 2007;5(11):1261–7.

44. Becker V, Vercauteren T, von Weyhern CH, et al. High-resolution miniprobe-based confocal microscopy in combination with video mosaicing (with video). Gastroint-est Endosc 2007;66(5):1001–7.

45. Kumagai Y, Monma K, Kawada K. Magnifying chromoendoscopy of the esoph-agus: in-vivo pathological diagnosis using an endocytoscopy system. Endos-copy 2004;36(7):590–4.

46. Pohl H, Koch M, Khalifa A, et al. Evaluation of endocytoscopy in the surveillance of patients with Barrett's esophagus. Endoscopy 2007;39(6):492–6.

47. Wilson BC. Detection and treatment of dysplasia in Barrett's esophagus: a pivotal challenge in translating biophotonics from bench to bedside. J Biomed Opt 2007; 12(5):051401.

48. el-Sharabasy MM, el-Waseef AM, Hafez MM, et al. Porphyrin metabolism in some malignant diseases. Br J Cancer 1992;65(3):409–12.

49. Regula J, MacRobert AJ, Gorchein A, et al. Photosensitisation and photodynamic therapy of oesophageal, duodenal, and colorectal tumours using 5 aminolaevu-linic acid induced protoporphyrin IX–a pilot study. Gut 1995;36(1):67–75.

50. Endlicher E, Knuechel R, Hauser T, et al. Endoscopic fluorescence detection of low and high grade dysplasia in Barrett's oesophagus using systemic or local 5-aminolaevulinic acid sensitisation. Gut 2001;48(3):314–9.
51. Georgakoudi I, Jacobson BC, Van Dam J, et al. Fluorescence, reflectance, and light-scattering spectroscopy for evaluating dysplasia in patients with Barrett's esophagus. Gastroenterology 2001;120(7):1620–9.
52. Zangaro R, Silveira L, Manoharan R, et al. Rapid multiexcitation fluorescence spectroscopy for in vivo tissue diagnosis. Appl Opt 1996;35:5211–9.
53. Ortner MA, Ebert B, Hein E, et al. Time gated fluorescence spectroscopy in Barrett's oesophagus. Gut 2003;52(1):28–33.
54. Perelman L, Backman V, Wallace M, et al. Observation of periodic fine structure in reflectance from biological tissue: a new technique for measuring nuclear size distribution. Phys Rev Lett 1998;80:627–30.
55. Wallace MB, Perelman LT, Backman V, et al. Endoscopic detection of dysplasia in patients with Barrett's esophagus using light-scattering spectroscopy. Gastroenterology 2000;119(3):677–82.
56. Backman V, Wallace MB, Perelman LT, et al. Detection of preinvasive cancer cells. Nature 2000;406(6791):35–6.
57. Kendall C, Stone N, Shepherd N, et al. Raman spectroscopy, a potential tool for the objective identification and classification of neoplasia in Barrett's oesophagus. J Pathol 2003;200(5):602–9.
58. Wong Kee Song LM, Marcon NE. Fluorescence and Raman spectroscopy. Gastrointest Endosc Clin N Am 2003;13(2):279–96.
59. Panjehpour M, Overholt BF, Schmidhammer JL, et al. Spectroscopic diagnosis of esophageal cancer: new classification model, improved measurement system. Gastrointest Endosc 1995;41(6):577–81.
60. Vo-Dinh T, Panjehpour M, Overholt BF. Laser-induced fluorescence for esophageal cancer and dysplasia diagnosis. Ann N Y Acad Sci 1998;838:116–22.
61. Panjehpour M, Overholt BF, Vo-Dinh T, et al. Endoscopic fluorescence detection of high-grade dysplasia in Barrett's esophagus. Gastroenterology 1996;111(1): 93–101.
62. Mayinger B, Horner P, Jordan M, et al. Endoscopic fluorescence spectroscopy in the upper GI tract for the detection of GI cancer: initial experience. Am J Gastroenterol 2001;96(9):2616–21.
63. Bourg-Heckly G, Blais J, Padilla JJ, et al. Endoscopic ultraviolet-induced autofluorescence spectroscopy of the esophagus: tissue characterization and potential for early cancer diagnosis. Endoscopy 2000;32(10):756–65.
64. von Holstein CS, Nilsson AM, Andersson-Engels S, et al. Detection of adenocarcinoma in Barrett's oesophagus by means of laser induced fluorescence. Gut 1996;39(5):711–6.
65. Brand S, Wang TD, Schomacker KT, et al. Detection of high-grade dysplasia in Barrett's esophagus by spectroscopy measurement of 5-aminolevulinic acid-induced protoporphyrin IX fluorescence. Gastrointest Endosc 2002;56(4): 479–87.
66. Bouma BE, Tearney GJ, Compton CC, et al. High-resolution imaging of the human esophagus and stomach in vivo using optical coherence tomography. Gastrointest Endosc 2000;51(4 Pt 1):467–74.
67. Poneros JM, Nishioka NS. Diagnosis of Barrett's esophagus using optical coherence tomography. Gastrointest Endosc Clin N Am 2003;13(2):309–23.

68. Evans JA, Poneros JM, Bouma BE, et al. Optical coherence tomography to identify intramucosal carcinoma and high-grade dysplasia in Barrett's esophagus. Clin Gastroenterol Hepatol 2006;4(1):38–43.
69. Qi X, Sivak MV, Isenberg G, et al. Computer-aided diagnosis of dysplasia in Barrett's esophagus using endoscopic optical coherence tomography. J Biomed Opt 2006;11(4):044010.

Medical Treatment of Barrett's Esophagus: Can It Prevent Cancer?

Richard E. Sampliner, MD

KEYWORDS

• Barrett's esophagus • Esophageal adenocarcinoma
• Proton pump inhibitors • Surveillance • Chemoprevention

The estimated new cases of esophageal cancer in the United States for 2008 were 16,470.[1] If a conservative estimate of the percent of adenocarcinoma is 60%, that translates into 9882 new cases. This is the most rapidly rising incidence cancer in the United States. The estimated deaths are 14,280, which reflects the lethality of esophageal cancer. It is the seventh leading cause of cancer death among men. The 5-year survival rate of esophageal adenocarcinoma in the United States is only 13%.[2]

The medical therapy for Barrett's esophagus (BE) can be conceptualized as reflux symptom control, surveillance endoscopy, and chemoprevention (**Box 1**). Gastro-esophageal reflux disease is the presumed background pathophysiology for the development of BE. As a group, patients who have BE have as much esophageal acid exposure as patients with severe erosive esophagitis.[3] Their anti-reflux barrier is defective, with long segment BE almost always accompanied by a hiatal hernia.[4] Although patients who have BE may have less sensitivity to esophageal acid exposure to the point that 40% of patients with BE have no bothersome gastroesophageal reflux disease symptoms,[5] the foundation of medical therapy is control of reflux symptoms. In the current era, that means proton pump inhibitor (PPI) therapy at a sufficient individualized dose to control heartburn and regurgitation. A proportion of patients requires twice-daily dosing. PPIs do not always control volume reflux, and patients still need to attend to not lying down after meals, especially large-volume meals. A high-calorie, high-fat, and heartburn-provoking meal may delay gastric emptying and necessitate more than 3 hours before lying down to avoid symptoms.

SURVEILLANCE

The value of surveillance endoscopy is controversial, and the intervals between endoscopies are based on impressions rather than evidence. At least in the United States, gastroenterologists accept the role of surveillance endoscopy and biopsy,

Arizona Health Sciences Center, Southern Arizona VA Health Care System, 3601 S 6th Avenue (111G-1), Tucson, AZ 85723, USA
E-mail address: samplinr@email.arizona.edu

Surg Oncol Clin N Am 18 (2009) 503–508
doi:10.1016/j.soc.2009.03.006
1055-3207/09/$ – see front matter. Published by Elsevier, Inc.

surgonc.theclinics.com

Box 1
Medical therapy of Barrett's esophagus

Proton pump inhibition

Surveillance endoscopy

Chemoprevention

---

although not necessarily following guideline recommendations. Current guidelines suggest that after two endoscopies 1 year apart lacking dysplasia, the interval of surveillance can be extended to 3 years.[6] Obtaining four-quadrant biopsies every 2 cm is the standard protocol. Ideally, each level should be in a separate container to track the location of potential dysplasia. Patients with long segment BE are notoriously underbiopsied, although the greater the number of biopsies the greater the likelihood of detecting dysplasia or early cancer in high-risk patients who have BE.[7]

If low-grade dysplasia (LGD) is detected, a repeat surveillance endoscopy in 6 months is appropriate to ensure that this is the highest grade of dysplasia present in the esophagus. An expert gastrointestinal pathologist should agree with the reading of LGD. The greatest interobserver variability in reading dysplasia is in LGD, and the greatest driver of increased frequency in endoscopy is the finding of dysplasia. An expert reading should decrease false-positive results and the unnecessary repetition of surveillance endoscopy. In the presence of confirmed LGD, annual endoscopy should be performed until no dysplasia is found on two consecutive endoscopies. If high-grade dysplasia (HGD) is read, again an expert must confirm this diagnosis. Any mucosal irregularity should undergo an endoscopic resection to have adequate tissue to be able to exclude the presence of cancer. A repeat endoscopy within 3 months with a four-quadrant biopsy every 1 cm is indicated. Confirmed HGD is a common threshold for therapeutic intervention—esophagectomy or endoscopic ablation therapy—depending on local expertise and patient preference.

The impact of surveillance endoscopy on cancer is supported by two database studies and many retrospective surgical series. In a community-based population study of esophageal and cardia cancer, 73% of patients whose cancer was detected by surveillance survived in contrast to no survival in patients whose cancer was detected without surveillance.[8] In an analysis of 777 esophageal adenocarcinomas identified in the SEER/Medicare database, upper endoscopy 1 year before the diagnosis was associated with earlier tumor stage and improved survival.[9] In five of six retrospective surgical series, survival of cancer found at surveillance was significantly greater than for cancer found without surveillance.[10–15] The average survival rate of the surveillance group was 84% ($n = 93$) versus 26% ($n = 366$) in the nonsurveillance arm (**Table 1**). Surveillance endoscopy seems to offer the opportunity for esophagectomy at a time in the course of the disease that offers better survival. Because these studies are not prospective randomized trials, lead time and length bias may account for the difference in outcome.

With the lack of randomized controlled trials, Markov modeling studies have been reported to assess cost-utility and the impact of surveillance on esophageal adenocarcinoma. The incremental cost-utility ratio for surveillance every 5 years was $98,000 per quality-adjusted life years gained.[16] The long interval derived from this modeling study has not been applied in clinical practice.

A Markov model was also applied to the prevention of esophageal adenocarcinoma (EAC) by endoscopic surveillance. Compared with no surveillance, the incremental cost-effectiveness of every-2-years endoscopy was $16,695 per life-year saved.[17]

Table 1
Retrospective surgical series of survival of EAC based on surveillance status

Author	Surveillance % (n)	No Surveillance % (n)	P Value
Streitz	62 (19)	20 (58)	0.007
Peters	90 (17)	20 (35)	0.09
van Sandick	86 (16)	43 (54)	0.0029
Incarbone	100 (12)	25 (85)	0.01
Ferguson	84 (12)	19 (68)	0.001
Fountoulakis	80 (17)	31 (74)	0.008
Mean	84 (93)	26 (366)	—

This finding suggests that endoscopic surveillance might be a cost-effective way to prevent EAC death. In modeling of screening and surveillance for BE, the cost-utility for surveillance of BE with dysplasia was favorable at $10,440 per quality-adjusted life years. In contrast, the incremental cost-effectiveness ratio of surveillance every 5 years in BE without dysplasia was cost prohibitive at $596,000 per quality-adjusted life years saved,[18] In another model not including patient preferences and assuming esophagectomy for HGD, surveillance for patients who had dysplastic and nondysplastic BE was cost-effective.[19] These various modeling studies highlight the need for higher quality data to inform our therapy of BE and more effectively prevent EAC.

ACID SUPPRESSIVE THERAPY

The standard medical therapy of BE is PPI and surveillance endoscopy. Can these therapies prevent cancer? There are no randomized trials of these interventions, but cohort studies and retrospective surgical series based on surveillance status support these strategies. In a meta-analysis of anti-reflux surgery versus medical therapy in patients who had BE, the esophageal cancer incidence was 3.8/1000 patient-years compared with 5.3 ($P = .29$).[20] Even assessing the last 5 years of this study, when PPIs were more likely to be used, there was still no difference (3.8 versus 4.2/1000 patient-years; $P = .33$). It seems that neither medical nor surgical anti-reflux therapy prevents cancer. The rationale for acid suppression was highlighted in vivo in a nearly decade old study. Patients with normalization of intraesophageal acid on PPI therapy had enhanced differentiation manifested by villin expression and decreased proliferation by proliferating cell nuclear antigen compared with patients with persistently abnormal esophageal pH.[21] Based on this study of intermediate endpoints as a surrogate for cancer in a small number of patients, intraesophageal pH monitoring and control have not been adopted in the clinical setting.

In a BE cohort study in the United States, 236 Veteran patients without dysplasia or cancer at baseline were followed an average of 5 years. The cumulative incidence of dysplasia was significantly lower in patients treated with PPI than patients on no therapy or H_2-receptor antagonists.[22] In a multivariate analysis, the use of PPI was associated with a reduced risk of dysplasia, hazard ratio 0.25 (95% CI 0.13–0.47; $P < .0001$).[22] In an Australian cohort of 350 patients who had BE with a median follow-up of 4.5 years, patients who delayed using a PPI for 2 or more years had a 5.6-fold (95% CI 2.0–15) risk of LGD compared with patients who used PPI.[23] The risk for developing HGD or cancer was similarly elevated: 20.9 (95% CI 2.8–158). These two cohort studies provide the strongest rationale for PPI therapy in patients who have BE (**Table 2**). In the clinical setting, in which only 10% of the diagnosed

Table 2 Impact of proton pump inhibition			
Cohort	n	Follow-up (y)	Impact
US	236	5	75% dysplasia reduction
Australia	350	4.5	5.6-fold increase LGD without PPI

patients with BE lack reflux symptoms, a randomized, placebo-controlled trial is not possible. A large trial in the United Kingdom has been initiated to compare low-dose to high-dose PPI in patients who have BE with an endpoint of cancer development.[24] The results of this trial should provide clinical guidance for PPI dosing in relation to cancer risk.

If BE is not diagnosed, needed therapy cannot be initiated. Because of many issues, including asymptomatic BE, access to care, and accuracy of endoscopic recognition, most cases of BE in the population are not identified. We are treating and surveying only the tip of the Barrett's iceberg. That approach minimizes any impact of therapy on neoplastic progression, which is diluted out by the large unrecognized pool not targeted.

OTHER THERAPIES

The evidence that standard medical therapy can prevent cancer is suggestive but lacks a strong evidence basis and is not conclusive, which has led to the concept of chemoprevention. The epidemiologic, in vivo, and animal model data are discussed. A systematic review and meta-analysis of nine epidemiologic studies assessed the association of aspirin and nonsteroidal anti-inflammatory drugs (NSAIDs) to esophageal cancer.[8] A protective effect was seen with any use of aspirin/NSAIDs and esophageal cancer odds ratio 0.5 (95% confidence interval [CI] 0.47–0.71). The impact on esophageal adenocarcinoma specifically was OR 0.67 (CI 0.51–0.87). Greater protection resulted from more frequent medication use.

With carcinogenesis in BE associated with increased cyclo-oxygenase 2 (COX-2) expression, COX-2 selective agents (Coxibs) have been assessed in an animal model and humans. In a rat esophagectomy model, a coxib and NSAIDs reduced the relative risk of cancer by 55% and 79%, respectively.[25] In a short-term human pilot study, a coxib reduced COX-2 expression and cell proliferation. A retrospective analysis of a large BE cohort study also demonstrated a significant reduced hazard ratio for EAC in current NSAIDs users.[26] Unfortunately, prospective trials to date have not had impressive results. In a randomized controlled trial of 58 patients who had BE and were using PPI with or without a coxib, only 28% of the coxib arm had decreased COX-2 expressions at 6 months.[27] Cell proliferation and dysplasias were not affected. In a larger randomized, placebo-controlled trial of a coxib in 100 patients with BE and dysplasia, there was no difference in the proportion of biopsies with dysplasia or cancer between the two arms.[28] Surprisingly, there was also no difference in prostaglandin and COX mRNA levels.

In the absence of convincing data from trials, medical decision analysis has been applied to chemoprevention. Because of the high risk of cancer in patients with HGD and BE, chemoprevention is cost-effective, with an incremental cost-effectiveness ratio ranging from $3900 to $5000.[29] An ambitious study in the United Kingdom that enrolled thousands of men who had BE is randomizing them to aspirin or no aspirin.[24] These patients are also randomized to high- or low-dose PPI. This study is proposed to demonstrate a chemopreventive effect of aspirin. A lower threshold than BE may be necessary to impact the development of cancer given the large unidentified population of individuals with BE (ie, patients with gastroesophageal reflux disease).

SUMMARY

Despite suggestive data, we cannot be confident that medical therapy for BE prevents cancer. Future research documenting the role of surveillance and the effectiveness of chemoprevention is awaited.

REFERENCES

1. Jemal A, Siegel R, Ward E, et al. Cancer statistics, 2008. CA Cancer J Clin 2008; 58:71–96.
2. Eloubeide MA, Mason AC, Desmond RA, et al. Temporal trends (1973–1997) in survival of patients with esophageal adenocarcinoma in the United States: a glimmer of hope? Am J Gastroenterol 2003;98(7):1627–33.
3. Champion G, Richter JE, Vaezi MF, et al. Duodenogastroesophageal reflux: relationship to pH and importance in Barrett's esophagus. Gastroenterology 1994; 107:747–54.
4. Cameron AJ. Barrett's esophagus: prevalence and size of hiatal hernia. Am J Gastroenterol 1999;94(8):2054–9.
5. Ronkainen J, Aro P, Storskrubb T, et al. Prevalence of Barrett's esophagus in the general population: an endoscopic study. Gastroenterology 2005;129:1825–31.
6. Wang KK, Sampliner RE. Practice parameters committee ACG: updated guidelines 2008 for the diagnosis, surveillance and therapy of Barrett's esophagus. Am J Gastroenterol 2008;103:788–97.
7. Levine DS, Haggitt RC, Blount PL, et al. An endoscopic biopsy protocol can differentiate high grade dysplasia from early adenocarcinoma in Barrett's esophagus. Gastroenterology 1993;105:40–50.
8. Corley DA, Kerlikowske K, Verma R, et al. Protective association of aspirin/ NSAIDs and esophageal cancer: a systematic review and meta-analysis. Gastroenterology 2003;124:47–56.
9. Cooper GS, Yuan Z, Chak A, et al. Association of prediagnosis endoscopy with stage and survival in adenocarcinoma of the esophagus and gastric cardia. Cancer 2002;95:32–8.
10. Streitz JM, Andrews CW, Ellis FH. Endoscopic surveillance of Barrett's esophagus: does it help? J Thorac Cardiovasc Surg 1993;105:383–8.
11. Peters JH, Clark GWB, Ireland AP, et al. Outcome of adenocarcinoma arising in Barrett's esophagus in endoscopically surveyed and nonsurveyed patients. J Thorac Cardiovasc Surg 1994;108:813–22.
12. vanSandick JW, vanLanschot JJB, Kuiken BW, et al. Impact of endoscopic biopsy surveillance of Barrett's oesophagus on pathological stage and clinical outcome of Barrett's carcinoma. Gut 1998;43:216–22.
13. Incarbone R, Bonavina L, Saino G, et al. Outcome of esophageal adenocarcinoma detected during endoscopic biopsy surveillance for Barrett's esophagus. Surg Endosc 2002;16(2):263–6.
14. Ferguson MK, Durkin A. Long-term survival after esophagectomy for Barrett's adenocarcinoma in endoscopically surveyed and nonsurveyed patients. J Gastrointest Surg 2002;6(1):29–35.

15. Fountoulakis A, Zafirellis K, Dolan K, et al. Effect of surveillance of Barrett's oesophagus on the clinical outcome of oesophageal cancer. Br J Surg 2004; 91:997–1003.

16. Provenzale D, Schmitt C, Wong JB. Barrett's esophagus: a new look at surveillance based on emerging estimates of cancer risk. Am J Gastroenterol 1999; 94(8):2043–53.

17. Sonnenberg A, Soni A, Sampliner RE. Medical decision analysis of endoscopic surveillance of Barrett's oesophagus to prevent oesophageal adenocarcinoma. Aliment Pharmacol Ther 2002;16:41–50.

18. Inadomi JM, Sampliner RE, Lagergren J, et al. Screening and surveillance for Barrett's esophagus in high-risk groups: a cost-utility analysis. Ann Intern Med 2003;138(3):176–86.

19. Gerson LB, Groeneveld PW, Triadafilopoulos G. Cost-effectiveness model of endoscopic screening and surveillance in patients with gastroesophageal reflux disease. Clin Gastroenterol Hepatol 2004;2:868–79.

20. Corey KE, Schmitz SM, Shaheen NJ. Does a surgical anti-reflux procedure decrease the incidence of esophageal adenocarcinoma in Barrett's esophagus? A meta-analysis. Am J Gastroenterol 2003;98(11):2390–4.

21. Ouatu-Lascar R, Fitzgerald RC, Triadafilopoulos G. Differentiation and proliferation in Barrett's esophagus and the effects of acid suppression. Gastroenterology 1999;117:327–35.

22. El-Serag HB, Aguirre TV, Davis S, et al. Proton pump inhibitors are associated with reduced incidence of dysplasia in Barrett's esophagus. Am J Gastroenterol 2004;99:1877–83.

23. Hillman LC, Chiragakis L, Shadbolt B, et al. Proton-pump inhibitor therapy and the development of dysplasia in patients with Barrett's oesophagus. Med J Aust 2004;180(8):387–91.

24. Jankowski J, Moayyedi P. Cost-effectiveness of aspirin chemoprevention for Barrett's esophagus. J Natl Cancer Inst 2004;96(11):885–7.

25. Buttar NS, Wang KK, Leontovich O, et al. Chemoprevention of esophageal adenocarcinoma by COX-2 inhibitors in an animal model of Barrett's esophagus. Gastroenterology 2002;122:1101–12.

26. Vaughan TL, Dong LM, Blount P, et al. Non-steroidal anti-inflammatory drugs and risk of neoplastic progression in Barrett's oesophagus: a prospective study. Lancet Oncol 2005;6:945–52.

27. Lanas A, Ortego J, Sopena F, et al. Effects of long-term cyclo-oxygenase 2 selective and acid inhibition on Barrett's oesophagus. Aliment Pharmacol Ther 2007; 26:913–23.

28. Heath EI, Canto MI, Piantadosi S, et al. Secondary chemoprevention of Barrett's esophagus with celecoxib: results of a randomized trial. J Natl Cancer Inst 2007; 99:545–57.

29. Sonnenberg A, Fennerty MB. Medical decision analysis of chemoprevention against esophageal adenocarcinoma. Gastroenterology 2003;124:1758–66.

Endoscopic Therapy in Barrett's Esophagus: When and How?

Stuart Jon Spechler, MD[a,b,]*, Raquel Davila, MD[a,b]

KEYWORDS

- Adenocarcinoma • Barrett's • Dysplasia • Esophagus
- Gastroesophageal reflux

There are two general types of endoscopic therapies available for the treatment of Barrett's esophagus: (1) endoscopic ablative therapy, which uses thermal, photochemical, or radiofrequency energy to ablate the Barrett's epithelium, and (2) endoscopic mucosal resection (EMR), in which a diathermic snare or endoscopic knife is used to remove a segment of Barrett's epithelium, usually down to the submucosa (**Fig. 1** A, B). After these endoscopic treatments, patients are given potent antireflux therapy (usually proton pump inhibitors) so that the injured mucosa heals with the growth of normal esophageal squamous epithelium rather than with the regeneration of more Barrett's epithelium.

The ablative therapies destroy metaplastic tissue, but do not provide a pathology specimen by which to judge the completeness of the ablation. In contrast, EMR provides large tissue specimens that can be examined by the pathologist to determine the character and extent of the mucosal abnormality and, for neoplastic lesions, the depth of involvement and the adequacy of resection. Although either type of endoscopic therapy can be used to remove nondysplastic Barrett's epithelium, most studies have focused on the use of endoscopic therapies for the treatment of dysplasia and early cancers in Barrett's esophagus.

USE OF ABLATIVE THERAPIES FOR BARRETT'S ESOPHAGUS WITHOUT NEOPLASIA

The thickness of nondysplastic Barrett's epithelium ranges from 0.5 to 0.7 mm, with a mean thickness of approximately 0.6 mm.[1] An ideal ablative technique would inflict an injury deep enough to destroy all of the metaplastic epithelium (ie, up to 0.7 mm), but not so deep as to cause serious complications like esophageal hemorrhage, perforation, and stricture formation. A number of endoscopic ablative therapies have been used to eradicate nondysplastic Barrett's metaplasia (eg, laser; multipolar

[a] Department of Medicine, Division of Gastroenterology, VA North Texas Healthcare System, 4500 South Lancaster Road, Dallas, TX 75216, USA
[b] Department of Medicine, University of Texas Southwestern Medical Center at Dallas, TX, USA
* Corresponding author.
E-mail address: sjspechler@aol.com (S. J. Spechler).

Surg Oncol Clin N Am 18 (2009) 509–521
doi:10.1016/j.soc.2009.03.003
1055-3207/09/$ – see front matter. Published by Elsevier, Inc.

surgonc.theclinics.com

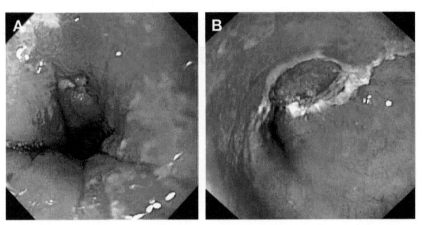

Fig. 1. (*A*) Endoscopic photograph showing Barrett's esophagus with a nodular, ulcerated lesion. Biopsy specimens of the lesion showed high-grade dysplasia. (*B*) Endoscopic photograph of the esophageal area shown in **Fig. 1** A after endoscopic mucosal resection using a cap-assisted technique.

electrocoagulation; argon plasma coagulation; radiofrequency energy; cold nitrogen gas; photodynamic therapy) but, so far, none has achieved the ideal of complete eradication of metaplasia without complications. In one recent study, for example, subjects who had Barrett's esophagus without dysplasia were treated with endoscopic ablation using argon plasma coagulation.[2] Nine of 51 subjects (18%) experienced transient side effects including chest pain, fever, and odynophagia, and five (10%) had a major complication including hemorrhage (two subjects), esophageal stricture (two subjects) and esophageal perforation (one subject). During a mean follow-up of 14 months, complete eradication of Barrett's epithelium was achieved in only 37 of the 48 subjects (77%) who had follow-up examinations.

Another recent study described promising preliminary results with a technique called banding without resection (BWR) for the ablation of nondysplastic, short-segment Barrett's esophagus.[3] The basis for this study was a serendipitous observation made by one of the investigators during a follow-up endoscopic examination for a patient who had variceal ligation performed for variceal bleeding. The investigator noted that a tongue of Barrett's epithelium, which had been overlying a varix banded one month earlier, was no longer visible. This suggested that the banding had ablated the Barrett's epithelium and, subsequently, the investigator initiated a study to explore the efficacy of BWR for the ablation of short-segment Barrett's esophagus. In a median follow-up period of 17 months during which subjects had a mean of three endoscopic sessions of BWR, complete eradication of Barrett's epithelium was achieved in 29 of 30 subjects (97%), all but one of whom had short-segment Barrett's esophagus. Adverse events included only mild chest pain and dysphagia that resolved within days.

Most studies on endoscopic ablation techniques for Barrett's esophagus have found that these procedures often leave visible, residual foci of metaplastic epithelium.[4–7] Partially ablated Barrett's esophagus can heal with an overlying layer of squamous epithelium that "buries" the metaplastic tissue and hides it from the endoscopist, and adenocarcinomas have developed from such buried metaplasia.[8] Partially ablated metaplastic epithelium also can develop new abnormalities in the expression of proliferation markers and tumor suppressor genes, raising the theoretical possibility that incomplete ablation of Barrett's esophagus might increase the risk of carcinogenesis.[9] Furthermore, even after apparent complete ablation, Barrett's metaplasia may recur over time.[10]

There has been much recent interest in the HALO[360] system (BÂRRX Medical, Sunnyvale, California), which uses a balloon-based array of closely-spaced electrodes to deliver radiofrequency energy to the esophageal mucosa. This system was designed with the intent of inflicting a uniform, circumferential thermal injury whose depth is controlled by a generator that can vary the power, density and duration of the energy applied. For patients who have Barrett's esophagus without dysplasia, treatment with the HALO[360] system leaves behind residual foci of intestinal metaplasia in approximately 30% of cases.[7,11] Noting this problem, the manufacturer recently has introduced a smaller, endoscope-mounted, radiofrequency catheter ablation device (the HALO[90] ablation catheter) that can be used for the focal ablation of metaplasia that remains behind after treatment with the HALO[360] system. By using a combination of the HALO[360] and the HALO[90] systems, a recent, uncontrolled study has described complete eradication of Barrett's epithelium in 60 of 61 subjects (98%).[11]

Although available studies have established the feasibility of endoscopic ablation for the eradication of nondysplastic Barrett's epithelium, it is not clear that the potential benefits of these procedures outweigh their substantial costs and risks. Barrett's esophagus per se causes no symptoms, and so the primary potential medical benefit of ablating nondysplastic Barrett's epithelium is the risk reduction of esophageal cancer. Modern studies suggest that subjects who have nondysplastic Barrett's esophagus develop esophageal cancer at the rate of only 0.5% per year.[12] No study has established that endoscopic ablation decreases that risk.

An evidence-based tool that can be used to help decide whether the potential benefits of a treatment outweigh its disadvantages is the calculation of the number needed to treat (NNT).[13,14] This is done using the formula NNT = 1/ARR, where ARR is the absolute risk reduction achieved by the treatment. Assume, for the sake of argument, that endoscopic ablation is highly effective and reduces the risk of cancer development by one-half, ie, from 0.50% to 0.25% per year. This represents an absolute risk reduction of 0.25%. Therefore, the NNT = 1/0.25% = 400. If this optimistic assessment of risk reduction attributable to ablation of Barrett's epithelium is correct, then 400 patients would need to be treated to prevent one cancer in one year. Such a large NNT might be acceptable for a treatment that is very inexpensive, safe, and convenient, but no endoscopic ablation technique meets all of those criteria.

One might argue that this estimate of NNT is unfair because it considers the number of procedures needed to prevent cancer for only one year, whereas a successful endoscopic ablation might prevent cancer for a lifetime. However, as noted above, metaplasia often persists or recurs despite ablation.[9] Thus, even an apparently successful ablation procedure may not confer lifelong protection from malignancy. Furthermore, the NNT calculation used in this example is based on a reduction of absolute risk that has not been established. It is not clear that ablation reduces the risk of cancer development at all, let alone by one-half.

In addition to reducing the risk of esophageal cancer development, another potential benefit of ablating nondysplastic Barrett's esophagus would be elimination of the need for lifelong endoscopic surveillance, with all of its attendant expense, inconvenience, and risk. As discussed above, however, the long-term benefit of ablation in reducing cancer risk has not been established, and the potential for cancer developing from buried metaplasia or from regrowth of Barrett's epithelium after ablation remains an unresolved issue. Without definitive data on cancer risk reduction, it may not be appropriate to terminate endoscopic surveillance after ablation of Barrett's epithelium based on the dubious assumption that the cancer risk has been eliminated. Thus, available data do not support the routine application of endoscopic ablative therapy for patients who have Barrett's esophagus without dysplasia.

USE OF ENDOSCOPIC THERAPIES FOR BARRETT'S ESOPHAGUS WITH DYSPLASIA OR EARLY ADENOCARCINOMA
Lymphatic Drainage of the Esophagus

When considering an endoscopic therapy for the treatment of Barrett's esophagus with dysplasia or early adenocarcinoma, the clinician should be aware of the extensive esophageal lymphatic system, which can serve as a conduit for the dissemination of neoplastic cells.[15] Unlike most hollow gastrointestinal organs, the esophagus has ample lymphatic vessels in the lamina propria. Therefore, even an intramucosal carcinoma has the potential to metastasize through these mucosal lymphatic vessels. The mucosal lymphatics drain into larger submucosal lymphatic vessels that extend throughout the length of the esophagus. There are also lymphatics in the muscularis propria that drain into larger vessels that traverse the muscular layers and adventitia of the esophagus. These two major groups of esophageal lymphatics, which intercommunicate with one another and with vessels supplying adjacent lymph nodes, provide the means for both longitudinal and lateral spread of esophageal neoplasms.

Endoscopic therapies, which ablate or remove only the esophageal mucosa, may not be curative if neoplastic cells already have disseminated through lymphatic channels. The frequency of lymph node metastases clearly increases with the depth of tumor invasion but, as noted above, such metastases have been found even in patients whose tumors appear to be limited to the mucosa. For patients in whom preoperative evaluations revealed only high-grade dysplasia or intramucosal adenocarcinoma in Barrett's esophagus, esophagectomy has revealed lymph node metastases in 0% to 7% of cases described in small surgical series.[15–19] For esophageal squamous cell carcinomas with a similar early T stage, interestingly, lymph node involvement appears to be more common.[19,20] It has been proposed that the reflux esophagitis associated with Barrett's esophagus may obliterate mucosal lymphatic channels and thereby prevent lymphatic spread of early esophageal adenocarcinomas.[19] Once an esophageal cancer breaches the muscularis mucosae to enter the submucosa, however, the frequency of lymph node metastases exceeds 20%.[15,16,19] With such a high frequency of lymph node involvement, endoscopic therapy is not considered definitive for patients who have tumors that involve the submucosa.

Endoscopic Ultrasonography for Tumor Staging

Whereas endoscopic therapy cannot be considered definitive for neoplasms that extend into the submucosa, accurate T staging is critical for patients who are to be treated endoscopically. Endoscopic ultrasonography (EUS) has been considered the most accurate, non-invasive diagnostic test for the T staging of esophageal tumors (**Fig. 2** A, B).[21] For early esophageal neoplasms, unfortunately, that accuracy is limited.[22,23] In one study of nine subjects who had esophagectomy for high-grade dysplasia or intramucosal carcinoma in Barrett's esophagus, for example, preoperative T staging by high frequency probe EUS was inaccurate in five of the nine cases.[23] EUS provided two false-negative diagnoses of esophageal cancer, one false-positive diagnosis of esophageal cancer, and two errors in tumor staging (one understaged, one overstaged). In another study of 15 subjects staged as having intramucosal adenocarcinoma by EUS, EMR specimens showed submucosal invasion in six (40%).[24]

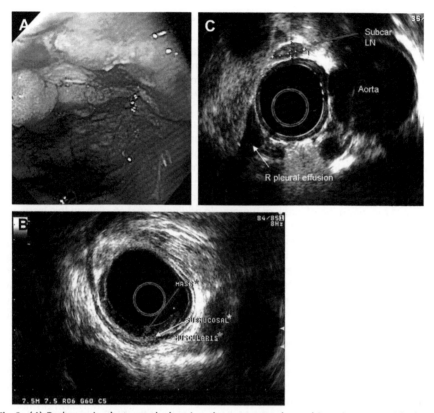

Fig. 2. (*A*) Endoscopic photograph showing the gastroesophageal junction area with short-segment Barrett's esophagus. Notice the nodular mucosal irregularity at 9 o'clock. (*B*) Endoscopic ultrasonographic image of the lesion shown in **Fig. 2** A. Notice that the hypoechoic mass does not extend into the hyperechoic, submucosal layer. The lesion was removed by endoscopic mucosal resection, and histologic evaluation confirmed that this was an intramucosal carcinoma. (*C*) Endoscopic ultrasonographic image from the same patient showing an enlarged subcarinal lymph node. Fine needle aspiration of the lymph node did not show malignancy.

The aforementioned study shows that histologic examination of tissue specimens obtained by EMR can be very useful for detecting submucosal invasion.[24] Another study in which the findings of preoperative EMR were compared with esophagectomy specimens for 25 subjects who had high-grade dysplasia or adenocarcinoma in Barrett's esophagus found perfect agreement between EMR results and findings at esophagectomy for tumor staging.[25] Therefore, EMR can be considered a diagnostic procedure for identifying submucosal invasion that might not be apparent by less invasive techniques like EUS, and a therapeutic procedure for eliminating dysplasia and early cancer provided there is no submucosal extension and no neoplastic cells are found in the margins of the EMR specimens. Although the accuracy of EUS for T staging is limited, EUS can add valuable information regarding regional lymph node involvement (**Fig. 2** C). If EUS reveals lymph node involvement that is confirmed by fine needle aspiration, then the patient has metastatic disease and endoscopic therapy alone cannot be considered definitive.

Results of Endoscopic Treatment for Dysplasia and Early Cancer in Barrett's Esophagus

When evaluating reports on treatments for dysplasia in Barrett's esophagus, it is important to consider the duration of follow-up. Patients treated for carcinomas traditionally are deemed cured if there is no evidence of recurrence at five years, because it is assumed that any cancer stem cells that survived the treatment would have become clinically manifest within that time period. As discussed above, however, patients who have high-grade dysplasia in Barrett's esophagus develop adenocarcinoma at the rate of only 4% to 6% per year. Consequently, it is not appropriate to conclude that the cancer risk has been eliminated for a patient who has no apparent cancer at five years after treatment of dysplasia. Unfortunately, the follow-up durations of most reported studies on treatments for dysplasia and early cancer in Barrett's esophagus are considerably less than five years, and this severely limits the conclusions that can be drawn regarding the efficacy of therapy. In addition, most studies on this issue are not randomized or controlled and most involve relatively small numbers of patients.

To date, photodynamic therapy (PDT) has been the most extensively studied of the ablative techniques for Barrett's esophagus. For PDT, patients are given a systemic dose of a light-activated chemical (usually a porphyrin or porphyrin precursor) that is taken up by the esophageal cells. The esophagus is then irradiated using a low-power laser that activates the chemical, which transfers the energy acquired from laser light to molecular oxygen. This results in the formation of singlet oxygen, a toxic molecule that destroys the abnormal cells and their vasculature.

In a multicenter, randomized trial of PDT using porfimer sodium for ablation of high-grade dysplasia in Barrett's esophagus, 138 subjects were randomized to receive PDT plus omeprazole 20 mg twice a day, and 70 received omeprazole 20 mg twice a day alone (without PDT).[26,27] No dysplasia was seen on repeat endoscopy in 77% of the PDT-treated subjects, and in 39% of the subjects who received omeprazole alone ($P < .0001$). During up to five years of follow-up, 15% of the PDT subjects developed cancer, compared with 29% of those treated with omeprazole alone ($P = .027$). There was no procedure-related mortality, but 69% of the subjects who received PDT developed photosensitivity reactions and 36% developed esophageal strictures that required dilation therapy.

In a recent uncontrolled study, 142 subjects who had high-grade dysplasia in Barrett's esophagus were treated with the HALO[360] system.[28] Twenty-four of those subjects (17%) had EMR performed before the radiofrequency ablation. There were no serious adverse events reported during 229 total ablation sessions, although one subject was found to have developed an asymptomatic esophageal stricture on follow-up endoscopic examination. At least one postablation endoscopy was performed during a median follow-up period of 12 months for 92 subjects, only nine of whom (10%) had high-grade dysplasia found in follow-up esophageal biopsy specimens. However, persistent low-grade dysplasia was found in another nine subjects (10%), and 42 subjects (46%) had residual foci of nondysplastic intestinal metaplasia in the esophagus.

The preliminary results of a randomized, sham-controlled trial of radiofrequency ablation for subjects who had dysplasia in Barrett's esophagus recently were presented in abstract form.[29] The trial included 64 subjects who had low-grade dysplasia and 63 with high-grade dysplasia who were randomized to receive either radiofrequency ablation with the HALO[360] system or sham ablation. Twelve months after the procedure, no dysplasia was found in esophageal biopsy specimens for 80% of the HALO-treated subjects who had high-grade dysplasia at baseline, and for 11%

of the subjects who received sham treatment ($P < .001$). For subjects who had low-grade dysplasia at baseline, 90% of the HALO-treated subjects had no dysplasia at 12 months, compared with 37% of the sham-treated subjects ($P < .001$). Complications were relatively few and easily managed. Five subjects developed esophageal strictures that resolved with dilation. One subject experienced upper gastrointestinal bleeding, and two developed chest pain following the procedure that resulted in overnight hospitalizations.

Although these reports have documented the feasibility of eradicating neoplastic epithelium with endoscopic ablation, they have not established the long-term benefit of the techniques for cancer prevention. Endoscopic ablation is expensive, and all of the treatments entail inconvenience and risks. Without histologic examination of the resected esophagus or durations of follow-up well beyond 5 years, it is not yet possible to verify claims that dysplasia and cancer are indeed "eliminated" by endoscopic ablation. A randomized trial has shown that PDT clearly is superior to omeprazole alone for eradicating high-grade dysplasia and for preventing cancer in Barrett's esophagus for up to 5 years, but the frequency of serious complications from PDT is disturbing, as is the fact that 15% of the subjects who received PDT nevertheless developed cancer within five years.[26,27]

Endoscopic Mucosal Resection

EMR can be accomplished by a number of endoscopic techniques, but much of the published experience involves a "suck and cut" method in which the endoscopist elevates the dysplastic area by injecting fluid into the submucosa, after which the elevated mucosa is suctioned into a cap that fits over the tip of the endoscope.[30,31] A polypectomy snare is then deployed around the suctioned area to remove it. A recent variation on this technique is the "band and snare" method, which uses a ligating device similar to that used for endoscopic variceal ligation. The device deploys elastic bands around the suctioned mucosal segment without the requirement for prior submucosal fluid injection.[32] The banded segment is removed using a polypectomy snare. The banding technique is quick and relatively simple (features that are major advantages if multiple EMR specimens are to be obtained at one session), and this technique has been shown to provide tissue specimens with depth and quality similar to those of the cap-assisted method.[33] Endoscopic submucosal dissection (ESD) is yet another EMR variation in which a diathermic, endoscopic knife is used to dissect a large segment of Barrett's epithelium en bloc.[34] Whichever method is used, EMR provides large tissue specimens that can be examined by the pathologist to determine the character and extent of the lesion, and the adequacy of resection.

Considering the depth and size of the tissue specimens obtained by EMR, there have been surprisingly few reports of serious complications (bleeding, perforation, stricture) and virtually no reports of procedure-related mortality.[30–47] However, esophageal stricturing may occur frequently if EMR is used to remove the entire circumferential extent of Barrett's epithelium in a single endoscopic session.[42,48] If the EMR specimen removes the neoplastic lesion and the margins of the specimen are negative for neoplastic cells, then the patient may be cured and an esophagectomy is unlikely to show residual tumor.[25] However, limited data suggest that a single cap-assisted EMR leaves neoplastic cells behind in the large majority of cases. In one report, for example, histologic examination of EMR specimens obtained by the cap-assisted technique from 88 subjects who had high-grade dysplasia revealed dysplastic tissue at the margins of the specimens in 72 cases (82%).[49]

The mean durations of follow-up in most reports on EMR for the treatment of neoplasia in Barrett's esophagus are too short for meaningful conclusions regarding efficacy in decreasing the incidence of cancer. However, the limited long-term data that are available are impressive. Ell and his colleagues[44] in Wiesbaden, Germany, performed EMR on 100 subjects who had early adenocarcinomas in Barrett's esophagus. The mean age was 62 years, and 69 of the 100 subjects had short-segment Barrett's esophagus. The cancers were early, meaning that the tumor diameter was less than 20 mm, the histology was well differentiated, there was no invasion of lymphatics or blood vessels, and there was no evidence of metastases, submucosal invasion, or lymph node involvement. EMR resulted in no serious complications, and the calculated 5-year survival rate was an extraordinary 98%. However, recurrent or metachronous cancers were found in 11% of the subjects during a mean follow-up period of 37 months. The recurrent tumors were treated successfully with more endoscopic therapy, but this high rate of recurrence shows that EMR often leaves behind cells with neoplastic potential.

A study from the Mayo Clinic confirms the observations of the Wiesbaden group.[45] The Mayo investigators compared long-term survival in subjects who had high-grade dysplasia who were treated either with esophagectomy or with a combination of EMR and PDT. There was no statistically significant difference in overall, long-term survival for subjects treated with either of the therapies, even though 6.2% of the subjects treated with PDT and EMR were found to have a metachronous esophageal cancer during the follow-up period.

A more recent report from the Wiesbaden group describes the long-term results of endoscopic therapies in a heterogeneous group of 349 subjects who had high-grade dysplasia or mucosal adenocarcinoma in Barrett's esophagus.[47] The endoscopic treatments included EMR alone for 279 subjects, PDT alone for 55, EMR and PDT combined for 13, and APC alone for two subjects. Serious complications of endoscopic therapy occurred in 5% of the 349 subjects and included important bleeding (two subjects) and esophageal stricture (15 subjects). During a mean follow-up period of 64 months, a complete remission (defined as complete elimination of the neoplastic lesion and at least one follow-up endoscopy showing no neoplasia) was achieved in 97% of the subjects. However, metachronous neoplasms were found during the follow-up period in 21%. Risk factors associated with metachronous lesions included long-segment Barrett's esophagus, multiple foci of neoplasia in the Barrett's epithelium, piecemeal resection of the tumor (a procedure generally required for larger tumors), time until achieving complete remission exceeding 10 months, and failure to perform ablation of the residual, nonneoplastic Barrett's epithelium after achieving complete remission. The calculated 5-year survival rate was 84%, and none of the deaths were from esophageal cancer.

These data suggest that EMR for dysplasia and early cancers in Barrett's esophagus is safe in experienced hands, and 5-year survival rates are excellent. However, most the studies have come from only a handful of highly specialized centers, and it is not clear that these results can be duplicated in a community hospital setting. Furthermore, recurrent neoplasms develop frequently after endoscopic therapy, especially if the residual Barrett's epithelium is not eradicated. Based on these findings, if endoscopic therapy is chosen for subjects who have dysplasia or early cancer in Barrett's esophagus, it seems reasonable to attempt to eradicate all of the Barrett's epithelium. After EMR, the residual Barrett's epithelium can be eradicated with an ablation procedure. Alternatively, EMR can be extended to remove the entire segment of Barrett's epithelium. Presently, it is not clear which of these approaches is preferable, nor is it clear which ablation procedure should be used and how long the EMR wound should be allowed to heal before performing ablation. One group found that EMR performed before PDT increased the risk of esophageal stricture formation,[50] whereas another group did not.[51]

RECOMMENDATIONS FOR ENDOSCOPIC TREATMENT OF HIGH-GRADE DYSPLASIA AND EARLY ADENOCARCINOMA IN BARRETT'S ESOPHAGUS

The Practice Parameters Committee of the American College of Gastroenterology recently has recommended that treatment for subjects who have early neoplasia in Barrett's esophagus should be individualized.[52] Treatment decisions should be based initially on considerations of age, comorbidities and life expectancy. Endoscopic therapy may be preferable to esophagectomy for an elderly and infirm patient who has an early esophageal neoplasm. The extent of the Barrett's metaplasia is also an important factor when considering endoscopic therapy. Is there short-segment Barrett's esophagus with a single focus of dysplasia that can easily be removed endoscopically, or is there a long-segment of Barrett's epithelium with multiple neoplastic areas that make endoscopic treatments difficult and less effective? In the latter situation, a young and otherwise healthy patient may be better served by esophagectomy than by endoscopic therapy. It is also important to consider the patient's preferences. Is the patient willing to accept the need for long-term endoscopic surveillance and the possibility of recurrence that accompanies the endoscopic treatments for neoplasia in Barrett's esophagus?

For patients whose endoscopic examinations reveal high-grade dysplasia or intramucosal carcinoma in Barrett's esophagus, we generally recommend EUS, primarily to seek and sample abnormal regional lymph nodes. If lymph node metastases are confirmed by EUS-guided fine needle aspiration, then endoscopic therapy alone cannot be considered definitive. EUS has very limited accuracy for T staging in this situation, however, and clinical management decisions should not be based solely on the results of T staging by EUS. In addition to EUS, extensive biopsy sampling of the entire segment of Barrett's epithelium should be performed to determine if there is multifocal neoplasia.

If endoscopy reveals any mucosal irregularity associated with the neoplasia, EMR should be performed to determine if there is submucosal invasion. Endoscopic therapy alone cannot be considered definitive if there is submucosal invasion. Even in the absence of submucosal invasion, a single EMR cannot be considered definitive therapy if there are neoplastic cells found in the margins of the tissue specimen. In this situation, additional treatment is required, although it is not clear whether that treatment should be further EMR or ablation.

Even if the margins of the EMR specimen are free of neoplasia, available data suggest that the residual, nonneoplastic Barrett's epithelium should be eradicated if possible to prevent the recurrence of neoplasia. Again, it is not clear whether that eradication should be effected by extended EMR or by endoscopic ablation. If all of the Barrett's epithelium is to be removed by EMR, it seems prudent not to perform circumferential EMR in a single endoscopic session, because this practice has been associated with esophageal stricture formation. For long-segment Barrett's esophagus, the combination of using EMR for the initial staging and/or treatment of dysplasia along with an ablation procedure for eradicating the remaining Barrett's epithelium seems most reasonable. With long-segment Barrett's esophagus, ablation will be easier and, perhaps, safer than circumferential EMR. Ablation should be delayed for approximately 2 months (the ideal interval is not known) after the initial EMR to allow the mucosal wound to heal. The preferred ablation procedure is disputed. PDT with porfimer sodium is the most extensively studied of the ablation techniques to date, but this procedure is associated with substantial inconvenience and frequent serious side effects. Preliminary data on radiofrequency ablation with the HALO system suggest that this technique may have similar efficacy to PDT but with less patient inconvenience and fewer side effects. Far more data are needed before dogmatic recommendations can be made regarding the choice of ablation procedure for the eradication of Barrett's epithelium.

REFERENCES

1. Ackroyd R, Brown NJ, Stephenson TJ, et al. Ablation treatment for Barrett oesophagus: what depth of tissue destruction is needed? J Clin Pathol 1999;52:509–12.
2. Manner H, May A, Miehlke S, et al. Ablation of nonneoplastic Barrett's mucosa using argon plasma coagulation with concomitant esomeprazole therapy (APBA-NEX): a prospective multicenter evaluation. Am J Gastroenterol 2006;101:1762–9.
3. Diaz-Cervantes E, De-la-Torre-Bravo A, Spechler SJ, et al. Banding without resection (endoscopic mucosal ligation) as a novel approach for the ablation of short-segment Barrett's epithelium: results of a pilot study. Am J Gastroenterol 2007; 102:1640–5.
4. Van den Boogert J, van Hillegersberg R, Siersema PD, et al. Endoscopic ablation therapy for Barrett's esophagus with high-grade dysplasia: a review. Am J Gastroenterol 1999;94:1153–60.
5. Sampliner RE. Endoscopic ablative therapy for Barrett's esophagus. Gastrointest Endosc 2004;59:66–9.
6. Bergman JJ. Latest developments in the endoscopic management of gastroesophageal reflux disease and Barrett's esophagus: an overview of the year's literature. Endoscopy 2006;8:122–32.
7. Sharma VK, Wang KK, Overholt BF, et al. Balloon-based, circumferential, endoscopic radiofrequency ablation of Barrett's esophagus: 1-year follow-up of 100 patients. Gastrointest Endosc 2007;65:185–95.
8. Van Laethem JL, Peny MO, Salmon I, et al. Intramucosal adenocarcinoma arising under squamous re-epithelialisation of Barrett's oesophagus. Gut 2000;46:574–7.
9. Garewal HS, Ramsey L, Sampliner RE, et al. Post-ablation biomarker abnormalities in Barrett's esophagus (BE): are we increasing the cancer risk? Gastroenterology 2001;120:A79.
10. Kahaleh M, Van Laethem JL, Nagy N, et al. Long-term follow-up and factors predictive of recurrence in Barrett's esophagus treated by argon plasma coagulation and acid suppression. Endoscopy 2002;34:950–5.
11. Fleischer DE, Overholt BF, Sharma VK, et al. Endoscopic ablation of Barrett's esophagus: a multicenter study with 2.5-year follow-up. Gastrointest Endosc 2008;68:867–76.
12. Shaheen NJ, Crosby MA, Bozymski EM, et al. Is there publication bias in the reporting of cancer risk in Barrett's esophagus? Gastroenterology 2000;119: 333–8.
13. Schoenfeld P, Cook D, Hamilton F, et al. An evidence-based approach to gastroenterology therapy. Gastroenterology 1998;114:1318–25.
14. Spechler SJ. Thermal ablation of Barrett's esophagus: a heated debate. Am J Gastroenterol 2006;101:1770–2.
15. Rice TW, Zuccaro G, Adelstein DJ, et al. Esophageal carcinoma: depth of tumor invasion is predictive of regional lymph node status. Ann Thorac Surg 1998;65: 787–92.

16. Feith M, Stein HJ, Siewert JR. Pattern of lymphatic spread of Barrett's cancer. World J Surg 2003;27:1052–7.
17. Oh DS, Hagen JA, Chandrasoma PT, et al. Clinical biology and surgical therapy of intramucosal adenocarcinoma of the esophagus. J Am Coll Surg 2006;203:152–61.
18. Peyre CG, DeMeester SR, Rizzetto C, et al. Vagal-sparing esophagectomy: the ideal operation for intramucosal adenocarcinoma and Barrett's with high-grade dysplasia. Ann Surg 2007;246:665–71.
19. Stein HJ, Feith M, Bruecher BL, et al. Early esophageal cancer: pattern of lymphatic spread and prognostic factors for long-term survival after surgical resection. Ann Surg 2005;242:566–73.
20. Siewert JR, Stein HJ. Lymph-node dissection in squamous cell esophageal cancer – who benefits? Langenbecks Arch Surg 1999;384:141–8.
21. Korst RJ, Altorki NK. Imaging for esophageal tumors. Thorac Surg Clin 2004;14: 61–9.
22. Falk GW, Catalano MF, Sivak MV Jr, et al. Endosonography in the evaluation of patients with Barrett's esophagus and high-grade dysplasia. Gastrointest Endosc 1994;40:207–12.
23. Waxman I, Raju GS, Critchlow J, et al. High frequency probe ultrasonography has limited accuracy for detecting invasive adenocarcinoma in patients with Barrett's esophagus and high grade dysplasia or intramucosal carcinoma: a case series. Am J Gastroenterol 2006;101:1773–9.
24. Larghi A, Lightdale CJ, Memeo L, et al. EUS followed by EMR for staging of high-grade dysplasia and early cancer in Barrett's esophagus. Gastrointest Endosc 2005;62:16–23.
25. Prasad GA, Buttar NS, Wongkeesong LM, et al. Significance of neoplastic involvement of margins obtained by endoscopic mucosal resection in Barrett's esophagus. Am J Gastroenterol 2007;102(11):2380–6.
26. Overholt BF, Lightdale CJ, Wang KK, et al, Internaup for High-Grade Dysplasia in Barrett's Esophational Photodynamic Grogus. Photodynamic therapy with porfimer sodium for ablation of high-grade dysplasia in Barrett's esophagus: international, partially blinded, randomized phase III trial. Gastrointest Endosc 2005;62: 488–98.
27. Overholt BF, Wang KK, Burdick JS, et al, on behalf of the International Photodynamic Group for High-Grade Dysplasia in Barrett's Esophagus. Five-year efficacy and safety of photodynamic therapy with Photofrin in Barrett's high-grade dysplasia. Gastrointest Endosc 2007;66:460–8.
28. Ganz RA, Overholt BF, Sharma VK, et al, U.S. Multicenter Registry. Circumferential ablation of Barrett's esophagus that contains high-grade dysplasia: a U.S. Multicenter Registry. Gastrointest Endosc 2008;68:35–40.
29. Shaheen NJ, Sharma P, Overholt BF, et al. A randomized, multicenter, sham-controlled trial of radiofrequency ablation for subjects with Barrett's esophagus containing dysplasia: interim results of the AIM dysplasia trial. Gastroenterology 2008;134(Suppl 1):A37.
30. Seewald S, Ang TL, Soehendra N. Endoscopic mucosal resection of Barrett's oesophagus containing dysplasia or intramucosal cancer. Postgrad Med J 2007;83:367–72.
31. Ahmadi A, Draganov P. Endoscopic mucosal resection in the upper gastrointestinal tract. World J Gastroenterol 2008;14:1984–9.
32. Peters FP, Kara MA, Curvers WL, et al. Multiband mucosectomy for endoscopic resection of Barrett's esophagus: feasibility study with matched historical controls. Eur J Gastroenterol Hepatol 2007;19:311–5.

33. Abrams JA, Fedi P, Vakiani E, et al. Depth of resection using two different endo-scopic mucosal resection techniques. Endoscopy 2008;40:395–9.

34. Yoshinaga S, Gotoda T, Kusano C, et al. Clinical impact of endoscopic submu-cosal dissection for superficial adenocarcinoma located at the esophagogastric junction. Gastrointest Endosc 2008;67:202–9.

35. Nijhawan PK, Wang KK. Endoscopic mucosal resection for lesions with endo-scopic features suggestive of malignancy and high-grade dysplasia within Bar-rett's esophagus. Gastrointest Endosc 2000;52:328–32.

36. Ell C, May A, Gossner L, et al. Endoscopic mucosal resection of early cancer and high-grade dysplasia in Barrett's esophagus. Gastroenterology 2000;118:670–7.

37. Buttar NS, Wang KK, Lutzke LS, et al. Combined endoscopic mucosal resection and photodynamic therapy for esophageal neoplasia within Barrett's esophagus. Gastrointest Endosc 2001;54:682–8.

38. May A, Gossner L, Pech O, et al. Local endoscopic therapy for intraepithelial high-grade neoplasia and early adenocarcinoma in Barrett's oesophagus: acute-phase and intermediate results of a new treatment approach. Eur J Gastro-enterol Hepatol 2002;14:1085–91.

39. May A, Gossner L, Pech O, et al. Intraepithelial high-grade neoplasia and early adenocarcinoma in short-segment Barrett's esophagus (SSBE): curative treat-ment using local endoscopic treatment techniques. Endoscopy 2002;34:604–10.

40. Pacifico RJ, Wang KK, Wongkeesong LM, et al. Combined endoscopic mucosal resection and photodynamic therapy versus esophagectomy for management of early adenocarcinoma in Barrett's esophagus. Clin Gastroenterol Hepatol 2003;1:252–7.

41. Conio M, Repici A, Cestari R, et al. Endoscopic mucosal resection for high-grade dysplasia and intramucosal carcinoma in Barrett's esophagus: an Italian experi-ence. World J Gastroenterol 2005;11:6650–5.

42. Soehendra N, Seewald S, Groth S, et al. Use of modified multiband ligator facil-itates circumferential EMR in Barrett's esophagus (with video). Gastrointest Endosc 2006;63:847–52.

43. Lopes CV, Hela M, Pesenti C, et al. Circumferential endoscopic resection of Bar-rett's esophagus with high-grade dysplasia or early adenocarcinoma. Surg Endosc 2007;21:820–4.

44. Ell C, May A, Pech O, et al. Curative endoscopic resection of early esophageal adenocarcinomas (Barrett's cancer). Gastrointest Endosc 2007;65:3–10.

45. Prasad GA, Wang KK, Buttar NS, et al. Long-term survival following endoscopic and surgical treatment of high-grade dysplasia in Barrett's esophagus. Gastroen-terology 2007;132:1226–33.

46. Larghi A, Lightdale CJ, Ross AS, et al. Long-term follow-up of complete Barrett's eradication endoscopic mucosal resection (CBE-EMR) for the treatment of high grade dysplasia and intramucosal carcinoma. Endoscopy 2007;39:1086–91.

47. Pech O, Behrens A, May AD, et al. Long-term results and risk factor analysis for recurrence after curative endoscopic therapy in 349 patients with high-grade intraepithelial neoplasia and mucosal adenocarcinoma in Barrett's oesophagus. Gut 2008;57:1200–6.

48. Rajan E, Gostout C, Feitoza A, et al. Widespread endoscopic mucosal resection of the esophagus with strategies for stricture prevention: a preclinical study. Endoscopy 2005;37:1111–5.

49. Lewis J, Lutzke L, Smyrk T, et al. The limitations of mucosal resection in Barrett's esophagus. Gastrointest Endosc 2004;59: AB101.

50. Prasad GA, Wang KK, Buttar NS, et al. Predictors of stricture formation after photodynamic therapy for high-grade dysplasia in Barrett's esophagus. Gastrointest Endosc 2007;65:60–6.
51. Yachimski P, Puricelli WP, Nishioka NS. Patient predictors of esophageal stricture development after photodynamic therapy. Clin Gastroenterol Hepatol 2008;6: 302–8.
52. Wang KK, Sampliner RE, Practice Parameters Committee of the American College of Gastroenterology. Updated guidelines 2008 for the diagnosis, surveillance and therapy of Barrett's esophagus. Am J Gastroenterol 2008;103:788–97.

Surgical Therapy for Barrett's Esophagus with High-Grade Dysplasia and Early Esophageal Carcinoma

Sébastien Gilbert, MD[a], Blair A. Jobe, MD, FACS[b],*

KEYWORDS

• Barrett's esophagus • Minimally invasive esophagectomy
• Outcomes • Treatment • Quality of life
• Esophageal adenocarcinoma • High-grade dysplasia • Survival

Esophagectomy has come a long way since the first successful attempt was described by Dr. Torek in 1913.[1] In the latter patient, the continuity of the upper gastrointestinal tract was restored using an extracorporeal rubber tube connecting the esophagus to the stomach. Today, esophagectomy is routinely accompanied by esophageal replacement with stomach, colon, or small intestine. It remains a complex operation requiring in-depth knowledge of the anatomy of the neck, chest, and abdomen. With continued improvements in surgical technique and perioperative care, esophagectomy will likely remain a viable option for the treatment of patients with Barrett's esophagus and high-grade dysplasia (Barrett's HGD).

BARRETT'S AND THE RISK OF ADENOCARCINOMA

Barrett's HGD is a marker of severe gastroesophageal reflux and chronic esophageal inflammation. Whether or not Barrett's HGD is a necessary precursor lesion to all cases of esophageal adenocarcinoma is debatable, and full discussion of this topic is beyond the scope of this article. Barrett's HGD and adenocarcinoma coexist in approximately half of esophagectomy specimens from patients with documented invasive adenocarcinoma, and in 0% to 72.7% of esophageal resections for Barrett's HGD.[2] After meta-analysis of surgical series of resected Barrett's HGD, the probability of invasive adenocarcinoma (12.7%) may be lower than once thought.[2] Because the

[a] Division of Thoracic and Foregut Surgery, Heart, Lung and Esophageal Institute, University of Pittsburgh, 200 Lothrop Street, Suite C-800, Pittsburgh Medical Center, PA 15213, USA
[b] Division of Thoracic and Foregut Surgery, Heart, Lung and Esophageal Institute, University of Pittsburgh Medical Center, 5200 Centre Avenue Suite 715, Pittsburgh, PA 15232, USA
* Corresponding author.
E-mail address: jobeba@upmc.edu (B.A. Jobe).

Surg Oncol Clin N Am 18 (2009) 523–531
doi:10.1016/j.soc.2009.03.008
1055-3207/09/$ – see front matter © 2009 Elsevier Inc. All rights reserved.

pathologic data from surgical case series is susceptible to selection bias, it may not reflect the true prevalence of esophageal cancer in patients with Barrett's HGD. Similar findings have been reported in patients who underwent endoscopic surveillance for Barrett's HGD. Their risk of developing adenocarcinoma is also widely variable (16%–56%).[3,4] In endoscopic surveillance reports, the incidence of cancer may vary because of differences in biopsy protocols and pathologic evaluations. When compared with surgical resection, only a small fraction of the Barrett's HGD mucosa is actually sampled during endoscopic follow-up (0.3%).[5] This may explain, at least in part, the observed difference in the prevalence of cancer between patients who are followed endoscopically and those who undergo surgical resection. Once invasive cancer has developed in association with Barrett's HGD, the patient is at risk for nodal metastases. Even if the probability of nodal metastases in early adenocarcinoma is relatively low, it has a major negative impact on overall prognosis.[6] The 5-year survival of patient with N1 esophageal carcinoma is uniformly dismal, regardless of the depth of tumor invasion.[7]

PREOPERATIVE EVALUATION
Cardiorespiratory Evaluation

In the United States, esophageal cancer patients are likely to be of male gender, over 50 years old, and diagnosed with comorbidity, such as obesity, hypertension, coronary disease, or diabetes mellitus.[8] Although noncardiac thoracic surgery is classified under intermediate-risk procedures for postoperative cardiac complications, esophagectomy is probably one of the higher risk operations in the specialty. Therefore, most patients being evaluated for esophageal resection will easily meet criteria for cardiac evaluation.[9] The guidelines recommend performing noninvasive cardiac testing only if the results will lead to a change in management of the patient. For patients with Barrett's HGD and no evidence of invasive cancer, it may be acceptable to delay esophageal resection until percutaneous or operative coronary revascularization has been achieved (3–6 months). However, in patients with invasive cancer, such a delay would not be recommended. Nevertheless, a routine pharmacologic stress test is important because it improves counseling on perioperative cardiac risk, and could potentially exclude surgery as a treatment option for some patients. Even if the evidence may not be uniformly supportive, careful consideration should be given to perioperative beta-blockade in esophagectomy patients, regardless of noninvasive cardiac test results.[10,11]

Pulmonary complications constitute the most common type of morbidity following esophagectomy.[8,12] Thoracotomy causes a significant decrease in forced vital capacity (35%) and forced expiratory volume in 1 second (FEV1) (60%) in the immediate postoperative period.[13] Although it is not an absolute necessity, obtaining pulmonary function tests before esophagectomy may help selecting a surgical approach and adjust postoperative care. For example, a patient with poor lung function may not tolerate single lung ventilation and may need early bronchoscopic intervention to clear airway secretions after surgery. Pulmonary function tests also provide additional objective data to estimate the risk of postoperative pulmonary complications. In general, patients who have a FEV1 or a diffusion capacity less than 40% of predicted are considered at high risk for postoperative pulmonary complications.[13]

ENDOSCOPIC AND PATHOLOGIC EVALUATION

Endoscopic ultrasonography (EUS) is a complimentary test to CT in the evaluation of esophageal cancer patients who are candidates for esophagectomy. It may provide useful information in cases where depth of invasion (T status) or lymph node involvement (N status) are used to guide neoadjuvant treatment protocols. On the other hand, EUS should probably be performed routinely in patients with Barrett's HGD, especially if a nonoperative treatment strategy is contemplated. In those patients, EUS has a reported sensitivity and specificity to detect cancer of 82% to 100% and 87% to 94%, respectively.[14,15] The false-negative rate approached zero but the false-positive rate was 13% in series where EUS results were correlated with esophageal resection specimens.[14,15] EUS can have a significant impact on clinical management, especially when a Barrett's HGD patient is found to have a previously undetected invasive cancer.

Finally, before submitting a patient to the potential morbidity and mortality of esophageal resection, the surgeon must seek confirmation of the diagnosis. This is an important issue in Barrett's HGD because of the documented interobserver variation between pathologists evaluating endoscopic biopsy specimens. A significant proportion of patients (up to 40%) may have their diagnosis of Barrett's HGD downgraded to low-grade dysplasia, indeterminate for dysplasia, no dysplasia, or no intestinal metaplasia once it has been reviewed by an expert pathologist.[5] Moreover, it may be equally difficult for pathologists to consistently and accurately distinguish Barrett's HGD from intramuscosal carcinoma.[5] Therefore, it is best to have dedicated gastrointestinal pathologists review biopsy specimens of all patients referred with the diagnosis of Barrett's HGD. In cases where pathologic review yields equivocal results, additional endoscopic biopsies should be obtained to devise an appropriate treatment strategy.

SURGICAL OPTIONS
Technique

Esophageal resections can be subdivided into two broad categories: transthoracic and transhiatal. Each category includes open and minimally invasive variants. The transhiatal approach mandates the creation of the esophagogastric anastomosis at the level of the neck, whereas the transthoracic approach adds the option to anastomose the stomach and the esophagus either in the left or right pleural space. Given the morbidity and potential mortality associated with anastomotic failures, prevention is of crucial importance. While the surgical literature is saturated with retrospective case series touting the superiority of one approach over another, there is a relative paucity of prospective randomized data to guide the esophageal surgeon. A meta-analysis of over 7,500 esophagectomy patients concluded that transthoracic esophagectomy may be associated with a 50% relative-risk reduction in anastomotic leak.[12] However, for anastomotic location, the prospective randomized data suggest that there is no significant difference in leak rates between a neck and an intrathoracic anastomosis.[16–20] The only trial demonstrating a difference has been criticized for including patients with substernal reconstruction, and patients who had a hand-sewn cervical anastomosis because of technical issues with the circular stapler.[21] As far as anastomotic technique is concerned, prospective randomized trials show no significant difference in anastomotic leaks between hand-sewn and stapled techniques.[22–27] Two of these six trials demonstrated a significant decrease in the rate of anastomotic strictures using a hand-sewn technique.[24,26] The additional time needed to create the anastomosis may be slightly shorter (9–14 minutes) when using a stapled technique.[22,27] The configuration of the gastrotomy needed to anastomose the esophagus to the stomach has also been evaluated prospectively.[28] The authors compared a generous (3-cm by 2-cm) crescent-shaped gastrotomy to a slit-like gastric incision and found that the former resulted in a significantly lower rate of anastomotic leaks after transhiatal esophagectomy (4% versus 20%). More recently, the use of a pedicled omental flap to cover the anastomosis has been evaluated prospectively.[29] Once again, investigators found that anastomotic leak rates could be reduced (3% versus 14%) by using this technique.

Beyond pure technical issues, retrospective reviews of large databases have identified a potential relationship between case volume and outcomes after esophagectomy.[30,31] In general, it has been stated that outcomes following esophagectomy improve when the hospital and surgeon volume is above a certain threshold. Unfortunately, a prospective comparison of outcomes between hospitals or surgeons with different case volumes has yet to be performed. It is definitely probable that, for most surgeons, experience and a constantly high-case volume will have a positive impact on perioperative outcomes. However, it would be an over-simplification in reasoning to develop a predictive model of surgical outcomes based on a single variable. Other potential factors (eg, skill level, surgical training, patient characteristics, outcomes in related procedures) may also affect postoperative outcomes significantly.

Outcomes

The outcomes of esophageal resection for Barrett's HGD and early esophageal adenocarcinoma are summarized in **Table 1**. To improve clarity and simplicity, only recent reports focusing on esophagectomy for Barrett's HGD have been included. The number of patients in the pathologic stage column is not always equal to the total study population because some Barrett's HGD patients were eventually found to have more advanced stage ($\geq$ IIa) esophageal cancers after esophagectomy. In the event that one institution published more than one case series, only the most recent data were included in the table. Most institutions used various surgical approaches to resect the esophagus. Follow-up time ranged from 12.6 to 59 months. In the series by Prasad and colleagues,[32] esophagectomy was compared with photodynamic therapy for the treatment of Barrett's HGD and early carcinoma. Although the survival was reported to be similar between groups, no specific percentages were provided. The specific rate of cancer recurrence in the surgical group was not provided but no patient died of cancer after esophagectomy. In the series by Chang and colleagues,[37] the overall survival was 88% at 46 months and there were no reported deaths from esophageal cancer. The 5-year overall survival published by Zaninotto and colleagues[42] was 79% for the entire group, and there was no difference between patients with Barrett's HGD alone and those with invasive cancer.

Only one series reported recurrence of cancer following resection of intramucosal cancer found within Barrett's HGD.[38] All other investigators reported no recurrence in that subgroup of patients. The weighted average recurrence rate for stage 0 and stage I or above esophageal carcinoma were 1.6% and 12.9%, respectively. The overall cancer-free survival was adversely affected by the presence of cancer within the esophagectomy specimen. While the majority of studies reported survival in excess of 95% for patients with Barrett's HGD alone, 5-year survival figures as low as 64% were published in patients with concurrent invasive carcinoma (see **Table 1**). The decrease in survival associated with the presence of invasive cancer provides support for surgical resection in Barrett's HGD patients who are operative candidates. The potential morbidity and mortality associated with esophagectomy constitutes the major trade-off for prolonged survival in these patients. According to the esophagectomy outcomes summarized in **Table 1**, the weighted average morbidity, anastomotic leak, and mortality rates were 33%, 2.8%, and 1.4%, respectively. Although the

Table 1
Outcomes following esophageal resection for Barrett's HGD and early esophageal adenocarcinoma

Author	n	Path. Stage (n)			Operation	Follow-up	Morb.	Leak	Mort.	Recur.		Survival		
		HGD	0	I						0	≥I	HGD	0	≥I
Prasad, 2007[32]	70	61	4	5	THE/TTE	59 mo	38%	0%	1.4%	—	NR	NR	NR	NR
Williams, 2007[33]	38	28	4	5	THE/TTE	32 mo	37%	3%	0%	0%	0%	100%	0%	0%
Peyre, 2007[34]	49	20	29	—	VSE	39 mo	35%	2%	2%	0%	—	NR	100%	—
Moraca, 2006[35]	36	11	11	12	TTE/THE	48 mo	44%	5.6%	0%	0%	14%	100%	100%	83%
Reed, 2005[36]	49	31	—	9	THE/TTE	56 mo	NR	4%	2%	0%	NR	100%	—	90%*
Rice, 2006[5]	111	59	40	6	NR	NR	NR	NR	0%	NR	NR	95%	77%	64%
Chang, 2005[37]	34	14	9	7	THE/TTE	46 mo	29%	3%	0%	0%	3%	NR	NR	NR
Westerterp, 2005[38]	120	13	41	76	THE	44 mo	NR	NR	4%	5%	24%	NR	NR	NR
Sujendran, 2005[39]	17	6	0	9	THE	32 mo	24%	17%	0%	0%	27%	100%	—	73%
Thomson, 2003[40]	18	6	5	7	NR	28 mo	56%	6%	0%	0%	0%	100%	80%	71%
Tseng, 2003[41]	60	42	—	13	THE/TTE	54 mo	29%	0%	1.7%	—	6%	88%	—	88%
Zaninotto, 2000[42]	15	10	—	5	TTE/THE	46 mo	53%	0%	0%	—	NR	NR	—	NR
Nguyen, 2000[43]	12	7	3	2	TTE(MIE)	12.6 mo	42%	0%	0%	0%	0%	100%	100%	100%

Follow-up period is median value; survival is survival from esophageal cancer.

Abbreviations: MIE, minimally invasive esophagectomy; NR, not reported; THE, transhiatal esophagectomy; TTE, transthoracic esophagectomy; VSE, vagal nerve sparing esophagectomy.

* Survival for stage I patients only.

morbidity rate may be similar to other series of patients with more advanced tumors, the leak rate and the postoperative mortality following esophagectomy for Barrett's HGD are much lower. Ideally, the surgeon should provide enough information for the patient to compare the risk of perioperative complications and the impact that coexisting invasive cancer can have on survival if not treated surgically.

QUALITY OF LIFE AFTER SURGICAL THERAPY

In order to remain a viable alternative to endoscopic therapies, the surgical community must continue to invest time and effort in improving postoperative outcomes and maintaining quality of life after esophagectomy. To the patient with Barrett's HGD, quality of life after treatment may be as or even more important than prolonged survival. In a pilot study, 20 patients with Barrett's esophagus were given a detailed evidence-based description of three treatment options: endoscopic surveillance, surgery, and photodynamic therapy.[44] The surgical option was an open esophagectomy with a quoted hospitalization period of 10 to 14 days, morbidity rate of 51%, and mortality rate of 5% to 10%. Seventy percent of patients chose endoscopic surveillance and 15% chose either esophagectomy or photodynamic therapy ($P<.05$). The most important concern about esophagectomy was the risk of postoperative death. It is unfortunate that this study did not include a larger number of patients. The patient preference may also have been related to the relatively high morbidity and mortality estimates provided as compared with recently published data (see **Table 1**).

In patients who have already undergone surgery, data on quality of life (eg, SF-36) show that the majority are not significantly affected by the lifestyle changes inherent to esophageal resection. Quality-of-life and performance-status scores appear to be preserved in 79% to 97% of patients.[32,33,35] The quality-of-life questionnaire scores were similar to the average United States population in the different areas tested (eg, physical functioning, bodily pain, vitality, and so forth).[37,45] However, the perception of one's health may be adversely affected by the diagnosis of cancer within Barrett's HGD.[45] Esophagectomy results in significant alteration in upper gastrointestinal anatomy and physiology (eg, resection of lower esophageal sphincter, denervation of stomach, pyloroplasty). Therefore, it is expected that a proportion of patients will experience some degree of heartburn, regurgitation, dysphagia, gas bloating, nausea, or change in bowel habits. If such symptoms were present before surgery, the patient may not report them because their occurrence is not perceived as a significant change from their preoperative state. This is an important reason why the surgical team should always attempt to elicit these symptoms from the patient to address the problem and to evaluate its impact on quality of life. Although it may be difficult or impossible to prove scientifically, the patient's decision to proceed with surgery will undoubtedly be influenced by his or her interaction with different physicians who may be biased in favor or against surgery. This situation will persist as long as there is conflicting evidence on the natural history of Barrett's HGD and its relationship to the development of invasive cancer.

According to the authors' interpretation of the literature, surgical resection remains the gold standard for staging and the best option for cure of early, often undiagnosed, esophageal carcinoma in the setting of Barrett's HGD. Given the lethal nature of invasive esophageal cancer and the significant probability of under-diagnosing malignancy, the authors still recommend esophagectomy for all operative candidates with Barrett's HGD. In discussions with patients, the authors focus on the elimination and potential prevention of invasive cancer rather than elimination of Barrett's mucosa. The authors do so because of published reports of recurrent Barrett's within the esophageal remnant after esophagectomy.[46,47] The data suggest that esophagectomy may not permanently eradicate Barrett's, and lend support to the use of routine surveillance endoscopies after esophageal resection. Finally, one of the most important objectives in the treatment of Barrett's HGD is to ensure that the patient has a clear understanding of the treatment options, both surgical and nonsurgical. Surgeons can achieve this goal by critically appraising existing therapies and continuing to explore new treatment modalities for Barrett's HGD.

REFERENCES

1. Dubecz A, Schwartz SI. Our surgical heritage: Franz John A, Torek. Ann Thorac Surg 2008;85:1497–9.
2. Konda VJ, Ross AS, Ferguson MK, et al. Is the risk of concomitant invasive esophageal cancer in high-grade dysplasia in Barrett's esophagus overestimated? Clin Gastroenterol Hepatol 2008;6:159–64.
3. Buttar NS, Wang KK, Sebo TJ, et al. Extent of high-grade dysplasia in Barrett's esophagus correlates with risk of adenocarcinoma. Gastroenterology 2001;120: 1630–9.
4. Schnell TG, Sontag SJ, Chejfec G, et al. Long-term nonsurgical management of Barrett's esophagus with high-grade dysplasia. Gastroenterology 2001;120: 1607–19.
5. Rice TW, Sontag SJ. Esophagectomy is the treatment of choice for high-grade dysplasia in Barrett's esophagus. PRO: esophagectomy is indicated for high-grade dysplasia in Barrett's esophagus. CON: surgery for Barrett's with flat HGD-No! Am J Gastroenterol 2006;101:2177–84.
6. Peters JH, Clark GW, Ireland AP, et al. Outcome of adenocarcinoma arising in Barrett's esophagus in endoscopically surveyed and nonsurveyed patients. J Thorac Cardiovasc Surg 1994;108:813–22.
7. Rice TW, Zuccaro G Jr, Adelstein DJ, et al. Esophageal carcinoma: depth of tumor invasion is predictive of regional lymph node status. Ann Thorac Surg 1998;65: 787–92.
8. Luketich JD, Alvelo-Rivera M, Buenaventura PO, et al. Minimally-invasive esophagectomy: outcomes in 222 patients. Ann Surg 2003;238:486–94.
9. Fleisher LA, Beckman JA, Brown KA, et al. ACC/AHA 2007 guidelines on perioperative cardiovascular evaluation and care for noncardiac surgery: executive summary. J Am Coll Cardiol 2007;50(17):1707–32.
10. Pennefather SH. Anaesthesia for oesophagectomy. Philadelphia: Lippincott Williams & Wilkins 2007;20:15–20.
11. Lindenauer PK, Pekow P, Wang K, et al. Perioperative beta-blocker therapy and mortality after major noncardiac surgery. N Engl J Med 2005;353:349–61.
12. Hulscher JBF, Tijssen JGP, Obertop H, et al. Transthoracic versus transhiatal resection for carcinoma of the esophagus: a meta-analysis. Ann Thorac Surg 2001;72:306–13.
13. Todd TRJ, Edwards ACR. Perioperative management. In: Pearson FG, editor. Thoracic surgery. 2nd edition. New York: Churchill Livingstone; 2002. p. 139–54.
14. Kinjo M, Maringhini A, Wang KK, et al. Is endoscopic ultrasonography (EUS) cost effective to screen for cancer in patients with Barrett's esophagus? Gastrointest Endosc 1994;40:205A [abstract].
15. Scotiniotis IA, Kochman ML, Lewis JD, et al. Accuracy of EUS in the evaluation of Barrett's esophagus and high-grade dysplasia or intramucosal carcinoma. Gastrointest Endosc 2001;54:689–96.

16. Walther B, Johansson J, Johnsson F, et al. Cervical or thoracic anastomosis after esophageal resection and gastric tube reconstruction: a prospective randomized trial comparing sutured neck anastomosis with stapled intrathoracic anastomosis. Ann Surg 2003;238(6):803–12 [discussion: 812–4].

17. Ribet M, Debrueres B, Lecomte-Houcke M. Resection for advanced cancer of the thoracic esophagus: cervical or thoracic anastomosis? Late results of a prospective randomized study. J Thorac Cardiovasc Surg 1992;103:784–9.

18. Hulscher JBF, van Ssandick JW, de Boer AGEM, et al. Extended transthoracic resection compared with limited transthoracic resection for adenocarcinoma of the esophagus. N Engl J Med 2002;347(21):1662–9.

19. Jacobi CA, Zieren HU, Muller JM, et al. Surgical therapy of esophageal carcinoma: the influence of surgical approach and esophageal resection on cardiopulmonary function. Eur J Cardiothorac Surg 1997;11:32–7.

20. Goldminc M, Maddern G, Le Prise E, et al. Esophagectomy by a transhiatal approach or thoracotomy: a prospective randomized trial. Br J Surg 1993; 80(3):367–70.

21. Chasseray VM, Kiroff GK, Buard JL, et al. Cervical or thoracic anastomosis for esophagectomy for carcoma. Surg Gynecol Obstet 1989;169:55–62.

22. Craig SR, Walker WS, Cameron EW, et al. A prospective randomized study comparing stapled with handsewn oesophagastric anastomoses. J R Coll Surg Edinb 1996;41(1):17–9.

23. Valverde A, Hay JM, Fingerhut A, et al. Manual versus mechanical esophagogastric anastomosis after resection for carcinoma: a controlled trial. Surgery 1996; 120:476–83.

24. Law SB, Fok M, Chu KT, et al. Comparison of hand-sewn and stapled esophagogastric anastomosis after esophageal resection for cancer: a prospective randomized controlled trial. Ann Thorac Surg 1997;226(2):169–73.

25. Laterza E, de'Manzoni G, Veraldi GF, et al. Manual compared with mechanical cervical oesophagogastric anastomosis: a randomised trial. Eur J Surg 1999; 165(11):1051–4.

26. Huguier H, Law S, Fok M, et al. Comparison of hand-sewn and stapled esophagogastric anastomosis after esophageal resection for cancer: a prospective randomized and controlled trial. Ann Surg 1997;226:169–73.

27. West of Scotland and Highland Anastomosis Study Group. Suturing or stapling in gastrointestinal surgery: a prospective randomized study. Br J Surg 1991;78(3): 337–41.

28. Gupta NM, Gupta R, Rao MS, et al. Minimizing cervical esophageal anastomotic complications by a modified technique. Am J Surg 2001;181:534–9.

29. Bhat MA, Ashraf Dar M, Lone GN, et al. Use of pedicled omentum in esophagogastric anastomosis for prevention of anastomotic leak. Ann Thorac Surg 2006; 82:1857–62.

30. Birkmeyer JD, Stukel TA, Siewers AE, et al. Surgeon volume and operative mortality in the United States. N Engl J Med 2003;349:2117–27.

31. Swisher SG, DeFord L, Merriman KW, et al. Effect of operative volume on morbidity, mortality, and hospital use after esophegectomy for cancer. J Thorac Cardiovasc Surg 2000;119:1126–34.

32. Prasad GA, Wang KK, Buttar NS, et al. Long-term survival following endoscopic and surgical treatment of high-grade dysplasia in Barrett's esophagus. Gastroenterology 2007;132:1226–33.

33. Williams VA, Watson TJ, Herbella FA, et al. Esophagectomy for high grade dysplasia is safe, curative, and results in good alimentary outcome. J Gastrointest Surg 2007;11:1589–97.

34. Peyre CG, DeMeester SR, Rizzetto C, et al. Vagal-sparing esophagectomy: the ideal operation for intramucosal adenocarcinoma and barrett with high-grade dysplasia. Ann Surg 2007;246:665–74.

35. Moraca RJ, Low DE. Outcomes and health-related quality of life after esophagectomy for high-grade dysplasia and intramucosal cancer. Arch Surg 2006;141: 545–51.

36. Reed MF, Tolis G Jr, Edil BH, et al. Surgical treatment of esophageal high-grade dysplasia. Ann Thorac Surg 2005;79:1110–5.

37. Chang LC, Oelschlager BK, Quiroga E, et al. Long-term outcome of esophagectomy for high-grade dysplasia or cancer found during surveillance for Barrett's esophagus. J Gastrointest Surg 2006;10:341–6.

38. Westerterp M, Koppert LB, Buskens CJ, et al. Outcome of surgical treatment for early adenocarcinoma of the esophagus or gastro-esophageal junction. Virchows Arch 2005;446:497–504.

39. Sujendran V, Sica G, Warren B, et al. Oesophagectomy remains the gold standard for treatment of high-grade dysplasia in Barrett's oesophagus. Eur J Cardiothorac Surg 2005;28:763–6.

40. Thomson BN, Cade RJ. Oesophagectomy for early adenocarcinoma and dyslplasi arising in Barrett's oesophagus. ANZ J Surg 2003;73:121–4.

41. Tseng EE, Wu TT, Yeo CJ, et al. Barrett's esophagus with high grade dysplasia: surgical results and long-term outcome-an update. J Gastrointest Surg 2003;7: 164–71.

42. Zaninotto G, Parenti R, Ruol A, et al. Oesophageal resection for high-grade dysplasia in Barrett's oesaphagus. Br J Surg 2000;87:1102–5.

43. Nguyen NT, Schauer P, Luketich JD. Minimally invasive esophagectomy for Barrett's esophagus with high-grade dysplasia. Surgery 2000;127:284–90.

44. Hur C, Wittenberg E, Nishioka NS, et al. Patient preferences for the management of high-grade dysplasia in Barrett's esophagus. Dig Dis Sci 2005;50(1):16–25.

45. Headrick JR, Nichols FC III, Miller DL, et al. High-grade esophageal dysplasia: long-term survival and quality of life after esophagectomy. Ann Thorac Surg 2002;73:1697–703.

46. O'Riordan JM, Tucker ON, Byrne PJ, et al. Factors influencing the development of Barrett's epithelium in the esophageal remnant postesophagectomy. Am J Gastroenterol 2004;99(2):205–11.

47. Wolfsen HC, Hemminger LL, DeVault KR. Recurrent Barrett's esophagus and adenocarcinoma after esophagectomy. BMC Gastroenterol 2004;4(18):1–5.

Role of Neoadjuvant Therapy for Esophageal Adenocarcinoma

Geoffrey Y. Ku, David H. Ilson*

KEYWORDS

- Esophageal • Gastroesophageal • Cancer
- Adenocarcinoma • Chemotherapy
- Chemoradiotherapy • Combined modality therapy

For locally advanced esophageal and gastroesophageal (GE) junction adenocarcinoma, surgery remains the mainstay of treatment. Various reviews have reported 5-year overall survival (OS) rates from 10% up to 30% to 40% with surgical resection alone.[1,2] For metastatic disease, chemotherapy alone results in response rates of only 20% to 40% and median survival times of 8 to 10 months.[3] Given the activity of these modalities, numerous studies have combined them in distinct neoadjuvant (preoperative) strategies for locally advanced disease. Contemporary multimodality approaches have included chemotherapy or concurrent chemoradiotherapy followed by surgery in an effort to improve the dismal prognosis of this aggressive cancer. Relatively few studies have focused on an adjuvant (postoperative) approach.

Currently, adenocarcinoma and squamous cell carcinoma histologies are treated similarly. For the purpose of this article, however, only studies that have enrolled adenocarcinoma patients are discussed. The results of these studies have been mixed, and their combined outcomes have failed to elevate any preoperative strategies to a clear standard for resectable esophageal adenocarcinoma. Recent trials involving preoperative chemoradiotherapy and pre- and perioperative chemotherapy have demonstrated improved survival over surgery alone, however. Based on these data, many clinicians treat locoregional disease with preoperative multimodality therapy.

NEOADJUVANT CHEMOTHERAPY

Despite the short-lived responses using chemotherapy alone in advanced disease, neoadjuvant chemotherapy is associated with many theoretical benefits.[4] This approach has the potential to assess tumor response to chemotherapy and direct the possible use of chemotherapy postoperatively or in the metastatic setting.

Gastrointestinal Oncology Service, Department of Medicine, Memorial Sloan-Kettering Cancer Center, 1275 York Avenue, NY 10065, USA
* Corresponding author.
E-mail address: ilsond@mskcc.org (D.H. Ilson).

Surg Oncol Clin N Am 18 (2009) 533–546
doi:10.1016/j.soc.2009.03.004
1055-3207/09/$ – see front matter © 2009 Elsevier Inc. All rights reserved.

Chemotherapy also may improve baseline dysphagia, downstage the primary tumor, and increase resection rates and treat micrometastatic disease that is undetectable at diagnosis. The large North American Intergroup 113 trial failed to show a survival benefit for perioperative cisplatin/5-fluorouracil (5-FU) plus surgery compared with surgery alone in 440 patients.[5] Patients in the combined-modality arm received three cycles of cisplatin/5-FU preoperatively and two cycles postoperatively. Pathologic complete responses (pCR) were seen in only 2.5% of patients receiving preoperative chemotherapy, and there was no improvement in the curative resection rate. The median OS rate was not significantly different in the two groups, and the 5-year OS rate with or without chemotherapy was 20%. The addition of chemotherapy did not change the rate of recurrence either locally or at distant sites. Outcome also did not differ by histology, with no benefit seen for preoperative chemotherapy for either adenocarcinoma or squamous cell carcinoma.

Renewed interest in preoperative chemotherapy was generated by a trial performed by the Medical Research Council Esophageal Cancer Working Group.[6] This study randomized 802 patients (nearly double the number of patients in the Intergroup trial) to surgery alone versus two cycles of preoperative cisplatin/5-FU. At a relatively short median follow-up of only 2 years, the chemotherapy-treated group demonstrated improved median OS (16.8 months versus 13.3 months) and 2-year survival rate (43% versus 34%). The curative resection rate was improved marginally from 55% to 60%, and the pCR rate was 4% in the preoperative therapy group. Results of this trial were recently updated in abstract form.[7] At 5 years, there continued to be a statistically significant but numerically smaller OS rate benefit for preoperative therapy (23% versus 17%).

It may be that the larger sample size compared with the Intergroup trial facilitated the detection of a small improvement with chemotherapy. A larger proportion of patients on this trial had adenocarcinoma histology compared with the Intergroup 113 trial (66% versus 54%). Two recent meta-analyses (described in detail later) suggested a potentially greater survival benefit from preoperative chemotherapy for patients with adenocarcinoma versus squamous cell cancer.[8,9]

Additional evidence to support the use of perioperative chemotherapy comes from the recent MAGIC trial performed in the United Kingdom.[10] This trial randomized 503 patients with gastric or GE junction adenocarcinoma to three cycles each of pre- and postoperative ECF (epirubicin/cisplatin/infusional 5-FU) chemotherapy and surgery or surgery alone. Perioperative chemotherapy resulted in significant improvement in 5-year OS rate (36% versus 23%). There was no improvement in the curative resection rate, however, and there were no cases of pCR. Because 26% of patients on this trial had tumors in the GE junction and lower esophagus, the results may apply to esophageal cancer.

Finally, data from the French FFCD 9703 trial of 224 patients with gastric or lower esophageal adenocarcinoma were presented recently.[11] Patients were randomized to two or three cycles of preoperative cisplatin/5-FU followed by surgery versus surgery alone. Patients who seemed to benefit clinically or radiographically from preoperative therapy or who had persistent T3 or node-positive disease at surgery also received an additional three or four cycles of chemotherapy. Preoperative chemotherapy was associated with a significant improvement in R0 resection rate (84% versus 73%), 5-year disease-free survival rate (34% versus 21%), and 5-year OS rate (38% versus 24%).

Although comparisons between different clinical trials must be made cautiously, the survival benefit seen with preoperative cisplatin/5-FU on this trial seems to be similar to that seen with perioperative ECF in the MAGIC trial. Because of the smaller sample size on this trial, however, outcome differences in as few as 10 to 15 patients would have changed the trial outcome. The trial also did not consistently stage patients with endoscopic ultrasound or stratify them by pretherapy stage. In a small-scale trial, even a slight imbalance in pretherapy stage might impact the trial outcome. Finally, a multivariate analysis indicated a greater survival benefit for patients with gastric versus esophageal primary tumors, which made the relative benefit of this therapy in patients with esophageal adenocarcinoma possibly less certain.

These data are summarized in **Table 1**. Overall, recent trials suggest a survival benefit for perioperative chemotherapy, although preoperative chemotherapy alone is associated with a low pCR rate and inconsistent improvement in the resection rate. Such a survival benefit also was demonstrated in a recent large, individual patient data meta-analysis of 12 randomized trials involving preoperative chemotherapy.[9] This meta-analysis revealed a 5-year survival benefit of only 4% with preoperative chemotherapy, with a suggestion of greater benefit for adenocarcinoma (7%) compared with squamous histology (4%).

NEOADJUVANT RADIATION THERAPY

Although trials that evaluated the benefit of preoperative radiation therapy largely have enrolled only patients with squamous cell carcinoma, a recent meta-analysis of five randomized trials that included a minority of patients with adenocarcinoma was unable to establish a significant benefit for preoperative radiation.[12] With a median follow-up of 9 years, an analysis of more than 1100 patients suggested a survival benefit of 3% at 2 years and 4% at 5 years that was not statistically significant ($P = .062$).

ADJUVANT THERAPY

Combined-modality therapy in esophageal carcinoma has long focused on preoperative strategies. The role of adjuvant therapy has not been studied extensively, and the data that are available suggest equivocal results. Again, many of these trials have exclusively treated patients with squamous cell histology.[13–15] An exception is a recent pilot Eastern Cooperative Oncology Group (ECOG) trial that evaluated four cycles of postoperative paclitaxel/cisplatin in patients with esophageal or GE junction adenocarcinoma.[16] Two-year OS rate was 60%, which is statistically superior compared with the historical control (38%, derived from Intergroup 113 trial). There also may be benefit from adjuvant concurrent chemoradiotherapy, as suggested by the results of the Intergroup trial 116 in gastric adenocarcinoma.[17] This trial revealed a significant improvement in overall and disease-free survival for the delivery of postoperative therapy with 5-FU/leucovorin and radiation compared with surgery alone. Because 20% percent of the patients treated had proximal gastric cancers (with involvement of the GE junction) and primary GE junction cancers, these data may justify the use of postoperative therapy in such patients who have not received preoperative therapy.

COMBINED NEOADJUVANT CHEMORADIOTHERAPY

Although recent pre- and perioperative chemotherapy trials have indicated a survival benefit, the low rate of pCR and the inconsistent improvement in operability have led researchers to investigate neoadjuvant chemoradiotherapy. Chemoradiotherapy typically involves regimens of cisplatin or mitomycin and continuous infusion 5-FU, with radiotherapy dosages from 30 to 40 Gy and up to 60 Gy in more recent trials. It results in pCR rates of 20% to 40%, with long-term survival rates of no more than 25% to 35%.[18,19] Superior survival is consistently achieved, however, in patients achieving a pCR to chemoradiotherapy (up to 50%–60% at 5 years).[20–24] These results are at

Table 1
Results of phase III preoperative chemotherapy trials in esophageal cancer

Treatment	Histology	No. of Patients	R0 Resection Rate (%)	Pathologic CR Rate (%)	Survival		Local Failure Rate (%)	Reference
					Median	Overall		
Perioperative cisplatin/ 5-FU + surgery	SCC (46%) + adeno (54%)	213	62	2.5	14.9 mo	3 y, 23%	32	Kelsen et al[5]
Surgery		227	59	N/A	16.1 mo	3 y, 26%	31	
Preoperative cisplatin/ 5-FU + surgery	SCC (31%) + adeno (66%)	400	60	NS	16.8 mo	2 y, 43% 5 y, 23%	13	Medical Research Council[6,7]
Surgery		402	54	N/A	13.3 mo	2 y, 34% 5 y, 17%	11	
Perioperative ECF + surgery	Adeno	250	69	0	24 mo	5 y, 36%	14	Cunningham et al[10]
Surgery		253	66	N/A	20 mo	5 y, 23%	21	
Perioperative cisplatin/ 5-FU + surgery	Adeno	113	87	3	NS	5 y, 38%	NS	Boige et al[11]
Surgery		111	74	N/A	NS	5 y, 24%	NS	

Abbreviations: Adeno, adenocarcinoma; bleo, bleomycin; CR, complete response; ECF, epirubicin, cisplatin, 5-fluoruoracil; etop, etoposide; 5-FU, 5-fluorouracil; N/A, not applicable; NS, not stated; SCC, squamous cell carcinoma.

the expense of significant toxicities—primarily hematologic and gastrointestinal—which have been greatest in trials using a higher dose of or twice-daily radiation or in which radiotherapy overlapped all cycles of preoperative chemotherapy.[25] The gastrointestinal toxicity associated with cisplatin/5-FU and radiation includes nausea, mucositis, and esophagitis, leading some investigators to mandate placement of enteral feeding tubes before treatment initiation.

The seminal phase III US Radiation Therapy Oncology Group (RTOG) trial 85-01 demonstrated the superiority of chemoradiotherapy over radiation alone.[26] This nonoperative study compared standard-fractionation radiation (64 Gy) to radiation (50 Gy) plus concurrent cisplatin/5-FU. The trial was stopped when data from 121 patients showed an improved median OS in favor of chemoradiotherapy (12.5 months versus 8.9 months). The 2-year survival rate was also improved in the chemoradiotherapy group (38% versus 10%), as was the 5-year survival rate (21% versus 0%).[27] Although most patients treated on this trial had squamous cell carcinoma, long-term survival was also seen in the small number of adenocarcinoma patients on the trial, with 13% of patients alive at 5 years.

In addition to a survival benefit, disease recurrence was significantly reduced by the addition of chemotherapy to radiation. At 1 year, recurrent disease was observed in 62% of the group that received radiation versus 44% in the chemoradiotherapy arm. Distant recurrence rates were 38% and 22%, respectively. The decreased local and distant recurrence rate suggested that chemotherapy helps to sensitize radiation and has systemic effects. Based on this study, chemoradiotherapy was established as the standard of care in the nonsurgical management of locally advanced esophageal cancer. Building on these results, alternative treatment strategies have been investigated. The RTOG 94-05 study compared a total radiation dose of 64.8 Gy versus 50.4 Gy during concurrent cisplatin/5-FU and failed to demonstrate superior results with the more intense regimen.[28] This study confirmed 50.4 Gy as the standard radiation dose when given in combined therapy with cisplatin/5-FU. The phase I/II RTOG 92-07 trial, which attempted to "boost" radiation with brachytherapy after external beam radiation, revealed significant toxicity, including a 12% incidence of treatment-related fistulas.[29]

PHASE III TRIALS OF CHEMORADIOTHERAPY

Four contemporary randomized trials have compared preoperative chemoradiotherapy followed by surgery versus surgery alone for patients with adenocarcinoma histology. A fifth trial, which reported no benefit for preoperative chemoradiotherapy, enrolled only patients who had squamous cell carcinoma.[30] The results are summarized in **Table 2**.

Urba and colleagues[31] from the University of Michigan randomized 100 patients to preoperative cisplatin/5-FU/vinblastine and radiation or to surgery alone. Despite a statistically significant decrease in the rate of local recurrence favoring preoperative therapy (19% versus 42%), 3-year OS rate trended toward improvement but was not statistically significant (30% versus 16%; $P = .15$). Rates of curative resection were equivalent in both groups (90%). Most patients treated on this trial had adenocarcinoma.

Walsh and colleagues[32] from Ireland randomized 113 patients with esophageal adenocarcinoma to preoperative cisplatin/5-FU/radiation or surgery alone. Rates of negative margin resection were not reported, although it was noted that the preoperative therapy group had a significantly lower incidence of positive lymph nodes or metastatic disease at surgery (42% versus 82%). A significant improvement in 3-year OS

Table 2
Results of phase III preoperative chemoradiotherapy trials in esophageal cancer

Treatment	Histology	No. of Patients	R0 Resection Rate (%)	Pathologic CR Rate (%)	Survival Median	Survival Overall	Local Failure Rate (%)	Reference
Preoperative CRT	SCC (24%) + adeno (76%)	50	45	28 (SCC 38%, adeno 24%)	16.9 mo	3 y, 30%	19	Urba et al[31]
Surgery		50	45	N/A	17.6 mo	3 y, 16%	42	
Preoperative CRT	Adeno	58	NS	25	16 mo	3 y, 32%	NS	Walsh et al[32]
Surgery		55		N/A	11 mo	3 y, 6%		
Preoperative CRT	SCC (35%) + adeno (63%) + other (2%)	128	80	16% (SCC 27%, adeno 9%)	22.2 mo	NS	15	Burmeister et al[34]
Surgery		128	59	N/A	19.3 mo	NS	26	
Preoperative CRT	SCC (25%) + adeno (75%)	30	NS	40	4.5 y	5 y, 39%	44	Tepper et al[35]
Surgery		26	NS	N/A	1.8 y	5 y, 16%	33	

Abbreviations: Adeno, adenocarcinoma; CR, complete response; CRT, chemoradiotherapy; N/A, not applicable; NS, not stated; SCC, squamous cell carcinoma.

rates was noted (32% versus 6%). Interpretation of this study is confounded by the poor survival of the surgical control arm (6% at 3 years), which is inconsistent with the approximate 20% or more 5-year survival rates reported for modern surgical series.[33] Other shortcomings of this trial include inadequate pretherapy staging that could have led to an imbalance in prognostic factors between both groups, the variable surgical procedures used, premature termination based on an unplanned interim analysis, and the relatively short follow-up period for surviving patients (18 months).

In a recent Australian trial, Burmeister and colleagues[34] randomized 256 patients to one cycle of preoperative cisplatin/5-FU and radiation or to surgery alone. Although the trial failed to show a survival advantage for patients who received chemoradiotherapy, they did have a significantly higher curative resection rate compared with the surgery-only patients (80% versus 59%). In this study, the administration of a single chemotherapy cycle may represent suboptimal delivery of chemotherapy. The pCR rate also was unexpectedly low in patients with adenocarcinoma (9%), perhaps also a reflection of the inadequacy of systemic chemotherapy administered on this trial.

Finally, results of the Cancer and Leukemia Group B (CALGB) trial 9781 were published recently.[35] This trial randomized patients to two cycles of preoperative cisplatin/5-FU and radiation or to surgery alone. Fifty-six patients were randomized before the trial was closed for poor accrual. Patients assigned to chemoradiotherapy had substantially improved median survival (4.5 versus 1.8 years) and 5-year OS rates (39% versus 16%) compared with patients undergoing surgery alone.

Overall, these randomized trials are associated with methodologic concerns, are significantly smaller than randomized preoperative chemotherapy trials, and produce conflicting results. They do suggest improved curative resection rates and decreased local recurrence. A survival advantage for preoperative chemoradiotherapy over surgery alone is not clearly demonstrated, although several studies suggested such a trend.

These observations are further supported by a recent meta-analysis, in which ten randomized trials of preoperative chemoradiotherapy versus surgery alone and eight trials of preoperative chemotherapy versus surgery alone were analyzed.[8] Preoperative chemoradiotherapy was associated with a hazard ratio of all-cause mortality of 0.81 versus surgery alone (95% CI 0.70–0.93; $P = .002$), which translated to a 13% absolute difference in mortality at 2 years. This benefit was irrespective of histology. Preoperative chemotherapy was associated with a hazard ratio of 0.90 (95% CI 0.81–1.00; $P = .05$) compared with surgery alone, which related to a 2-year absolute survival benefit of 7%. Although there was a benefit for patients with adenocarcinoma histology (hazard ratio 0.78; 95% CI 0.64–0.95; $P = .014$), there did not seem to be any benefit of preoperative chemotherapy for patients with squamous histology (hazard ratio 0.88; 95% CI 0.75–1.03; $P = .12$).

The possible superiority of preoperative chemoradiotherapy over preoperative chemotherapy also was suggested by a randomized study recently presented in abstract form.[36] In this study by Stahl and colleagues for the German Esophageal Cancer Study Group, patients were randomized to preoperative chemotherapy with cisplatin/5-FU/leucovorin followed by surgery versus cisplatin/5-FU/leucovorin followed by chemoradiotherapy with cisplatin/etoposide and then surgery. One hundred twenty eligible patients were randomized before the trial was closed because of poor accrual. The results revealed a trend toward improved local progression-free survival rate (77% versus 59%), median OS (32.8 versus 21.1 months), and 3-year survival rate (43% versus 27%) for the chemoradiotherapy over chemotherapy group, but these results were not statistically significant ($P = .14$). The pCR rate (16% versus 2%) and node-negative status (64% versus 37%) were significantly higher in the chemoradiotherapy group. Strengths of this trial include the careful pretherapy staging (which included endoscopic ultrasound and laparoscopy), the enrollment only of high-risk patients with at least T3 or node-positive tumors, and the careful balancing of pretherapy stage between the two treatment arms.

DEFINITIVE CHEMORADIOTHERAPY WITHOUT SURGERY

The question of whether there is a survival benefit for surgery after chemoradiotherapy has not been answered definitively for esophageal adenocarcinoma. Although two recent randomized trials compared definitive chemoradiotherapy versus chemoradiotherapy followed by surgery, one trial exclusively enrolled patients with squamous cell carcinoma,[22] whereas only approximately 10% of patients on the other trial had adenocarcinoma histology.[37] Incidentally, neither of these trials demonstrated a survival benefit for chemoradiotherapy after surgery in this group composed mostly of patients with squamous cell cancer. Local control seemed to have been improved, albeit at the cost of increased treatment-related mortality in the surgery groups.

As a related issue, definitive chemoradiotherapy alone versus surgery alone was recently compared in a Scandinavian phase III trial of 91 patients who were randomized to receive either cisplatin/5-FU and radiation alone or surgery.[38] At a median follow-up of 51.8 months, there was no survival difference between both groups. Although this study may be underpowered to detect small survival differences, the data suggested that definitive chemoradiotherapy is an acceptable approach for patients who have contraindications to surgery.

NEWER CHEMORADIOTHERAPY REGIMENS

The poor results and toxicity of therapy obtained with conventional cisplatin/5-FU–based regimens have led to the search for more effective and better tolerated regimens. Paclitaxel-based chemotherapy has undergone extensive evaluation in combined modality therapy trials with radiation. These phase II trials have combined a conventional schedule of paclitaxel/cisplatin every 3 weeks,[39,40] weekly paclitaxel with cisplatin every 3 weeks[41] or weekly paclitaxel with weekly cisplatin[42,43] or with weekly carboplatin.[44] They have reported pCR rates of 19% to 46%, with toxicities generally less in trials with weekly chemotherapy regimens. Consistently, pCR rates in recent trials are higher in patients with squamous cancer compared with patients with adenocarcinoma histology.[34]

Other trials have combined paclitaxel and continuous infusion 5-FU and cisplatin or carboplatin.[45–48] These three-drug trials have reported substantial toxicities, including severe myelosuppression and esophagitis, but have not consistently demonstrated superior results. Retrospective data from the Massachusetts General Hospital indicated similar pCR rates and 3-year survival for a three-drug regimen of paclitaxel/cisplatin/5-FU and radiation compared with cisplatin/5-FU and radiation.[49] The relative efficacy and toxicity of paclitaxel-based chemotherapy will be answered in the recently completed RTOG trial 0113. In this trial, a regimen of weekly paclitaxel/cisplatin and radiation was compared with weekly paclitaxel/5-FU and radiation in locally advanced esophageal cancer, as definitive therapy without surgery.

Irinotecan-based regimens also have been investigated. Based on activity observed in the metastatic setting,[50] a regimen of weekly irinotecan/cisplatin and radiation has been evaluated in phase I and II studies.[51–53] The regimen was found to be tolerable and is associated with pCR rates of 19% to 35%. Based on these positive results, the CALGB 80302 trial is currently evaluating weekly irinotecan/cisplatin with concurrent radiation for locally advanced esophageal cancer.

The relative efficacy and toxicity of paclitaxel-based chemotherapy was recently compared in the randomized phase II RTOG trial 0113, where a regimen of induction paclitaxel/5-FU/cisplatin followed by weekly paclitaxel/5-FU and radiation was compared to induction paclitaxel/cisplatin and weekly paclitaxel/cisplatin with radiation as definitive therapy in locally advanced disease.[54] Neither arm achieved the pre-specified 1-year survival rate, although there appeared to be a non-significant trend towards improved survival in the 5-FU-containing arm (median OS 29 versus 15 months). Both arms were also associated with a grade 3/4 toxicity rate of >80%. The authors concluded that neither arm was sufficiently superior to historical cisplatin/5-FU and radiation to warrant further investigation.

Although beyond the scope of this article, targeted therapies are also undergoing evaluation as part of newer regimens in phase III trials. In the United Kingdom, the MAGIC-B trial is randomizing patients with locally advanced gastric and GE junction cancer to perioperative epirubicin/cisplatin/capecitabine chemotherapy with or without bevacizumab, a monoclonal antibody against vascular endothelial growth factor. The RTOG 0436 trial is evaluating cisplatin/paclitaxel and radiation with or without cetuximab, a monoclonal antibody against epidermal growth factor receptor, in the nonoperative management of esophageal cancer.

POSITRON EMISSION TOMOGRAPHY–DIRECTED THERAPY

[^{18}F]2-fluoro-deoxy-D-glucose positron emission tomography (FDG-PET) scanning is emerging as an important tool to investigate response to therapy. Several studies have demonstrated that the degree of response detected by PET after preoperative chemoradiotherapy[55,56] or chemotherapy[57,58] is highly correlated with pathologic response at surgery and patient survival.

The German MUNICON trial evaluated the strategy of taking patients with locally advanced GE junction tumors with a suboptimal response to 2 weeks of induction chemotherapy with cisplatin/5-FU—as determined by serial PET scans—directly to immediate surgery, instead of continuing with presumably ineffective chemotherapy. Patients with a metabolic response by PET (defined as $\geq$ 35% reduction in standard uptake value between baseline and repeat PET scan) continued with an additional 12 weeks of chemotherapy before surgery.[59] This trial revealed a significantly improved R0 resection rate (96% versus 74%), major pathologic response rate (58% versus 0%), median event-free survival (29.7 versus 14.1 months), and median OS (median not reached versus 25.8 months) for PET responders versus PET nonresponders. The outcome for PET nonresponders referred for immediate surgery was similar to the outcome of such patients in an earlier trial who completed 3 months of preoperative chemotherapy,[57] indicating that nonresponding patients were not compromised by referral to immediate surgery.

Building on the results of the MUNICON trial, the same investigators recently reported the results of the MUNICON-2 trial in abstract form.[60] In this variant trial design, PET nonresponders to induction 5-FU/cisplatin were treated with "salvage" chemoradiotherapy with cisplatin before surgery. When compared with the PET responders who completed 3 months of 5-FU/cisplatin before surgery, the PET nonresponders had an inferior pCR rate (0% versus 16%), a higher R1/R2 resection rate (31% versus 16%), and an inferior 1-year progression-free survival rate (46% versus 63%). These results are not entirely surprising, given the use of chemotherapy during concurrent radiation that was assessed to be suboptimal by PET when administered as induction therapy.

Based on the poor outcome of PET nonresponders in these studies, another promising strategy would be to use PET assessment after induction chemotherapy to dictate chemotherapy during concurrent radiation. Responding patients can continue with the same chemotherapy regimen during concurrent radiation, whereas nonresponding patients can be switched to alternative, non–cross-resistant chemotherapy during radiation. Long-term disease-free survival has been reported in patients who progressed on induction chemotherapy but were changed to alternative chemotherapy during subsequent combined chemoradiotherapy.[53]

SUMMARY

The treatment of esophageal and GE junction adenocarcinoma remains a great challenge to medical, surgical, and radiation oncologists. Recent trials indicate that more than surgery alone should be offered to patients. Primary chemoradiotherapy is currently the standard of care in the treatment of inoperable, localized disease. The use of preoperative chemoradiotherapy continues to be investigated but seems to lead to improved OS in patients who have had a pCR. Several recent trials suggested that perioperative chemotherapy is also a valid strategy. For patients undergoing primary resection of lower esophageal/GE junction adenocarcinoma, postoperative chemoradiotherapy also seems to improve survival compared with surgery alone.

Although surgery remains the standard curative treatment for early-stage disease, there are data that definitive chemoradiotherapy results in similar survival rates as surgery alone. Unlike in squamous cell carcinoma, there are currently inadequate data to determine if patients with adenocarcinoma who respond to initial chemoradiotherapy derive a survival benefit from subsequent surgery. Finally, the development and evaluation of new chemotherapy regimens, the incorporation of targeted biologic agents, and the use of sensitive metabolic imaging to assess response to therapy represent future directions for the improved treatment of esophageal cancer.

REFERENCES

1. Muller JM, Erasmi H, Stelzner M, et al. Surgical therapy of oesophageal carcinoma. Br J Surg 1990;77:845–57.
2. Hulscher JB, van Sandick JW, de Boer AG, et al. Extended transthoracic resection compared with limited transhiatal resection for adenocarcinoma of the esophagus. N Engl J Med 2002;347:1662–9.
3. Enzinger PC, Mayer RJ. Esophageal cancer. N Engl J Med 2003;349:2241–52.
4. Harris DT, Mastrangelo MJ. Theory and application of early systemic therapy. Semin Oncol 1991;18:493–503.
5. Kelsen DP, Ginsberg R, Pajak TF, et al. Chemotherapy followed by surgery compared with surgery alone for localized esophageal cancer. N Engl J Med 1998;339:1979–84.
6. Medical Research Council Oesophageal Cancer Working Group. Surgical resection with or without preoperative chemotherapy in oesophageal cancer: a randomised controlled trial. Lancet 2002;359:1727–33.
7. Allum W, Fogarty P, Stenning S, et al. Long term results of the MRC OEO2 randomized trial of surgery with or without preoperative chemotherapy in resectable esophageal cancer [abstract 9]. Proceedings of the Gastrointestinals American Society of Clinical Oncologists 2008.
8. Gebski V, Burmeister B, Smithers BM, et al. Survival benefits from neoadjuvant chemoradiotherapy or chemotherapy in oesophageal carcinoma: a meta-analysis. Lancet Oncol 2007;8:226–34.

9. Thirion P, Michiels S, Le Maître A, et al. Individual patient data-based meta-analysis assessing pre-operative chemotherapy in resectable oesophageal carcinoma [abstract 4512]. In: J Clin Oncol 2007;25:18S.

10. Cunningham D, Allum WH, Stenning SP, et al. Perioperative chemotherapy versus surgery alone for resectable gastroesophageal cancer. N Engl J Med 2006;355: 11–20.

11. Boige V, Pignon J, Saint-Aubert B, et al. Final results of a randomized trial comparing preoperative 5-fluorouracil (F)/cisplatin (P) to surgery alone in adenocarcinoma of stomach and lower esophagus (ASLE): FNLCC ACCORD07-FFCD 9703 trial [abstract 4510]. J Clin Oncol 2007;25:18S.

12. Arnott SJ, Duncan W, Gignoux M, et al. Preoperative radiotherapy for esophageal carcinoma. Cochrane Database Syst Rev 2005:CD001799.

13. Ando N, Iizuka T, Ide H, et al. Surgery plus chemotherapy compared with surgery alone for localized squamous cell carcinoma of the thoracic esophagus: a Japan Clinical Oncology Group Study–JCOG9204. J Clin Oncol 2003;21:4592–6.

14. Ando N, Iizuka T, Kakegawa T, et al. A randomized trial of surgery with and without chemotherapy for localized squamous carcinoma of the thoracic esophagus: the Japan Clinical Oncology Group Study. J Thorac Cardiovasc Surg 1997; 114:205–9.

15. Pouliquen X, Levard H, Hay JM, et al. 5-Fluorouracil and cisplatin therapy after palliative surgical resection of squamous cell carcinoma of the esophagus: a multicenter randomized trial. French Associations for Surgical Research. Ann Surg 1996;223:127–33.

16. Armanios M, Xu R, Forastiere AA, et al. Adjuvant chemotherapy for resected adenocarcinoma of the esophagus, gastro-esophageal junction, and cardia: phase II trial (E8296) of the Eastern Cooperative Oncology Group. J Clin Oncol 2004;22:4495–9.

17. Macdonald JS, Smalley SR, Benedetti J, et al. Chemoradiotherapy after surgery compared with surgery alone for adenocarcinoma of the stomach or gastroesophageal junction. N Engl J Med 2001;345:725–30.

18. Coia LR, Engstrom PF, Paul AR, et al. Long-term results of infusional 5-FU, mitomycin-C and radiation as primary management of esophageal carcinoma. Int J Radiat Oncol Biol Phys 1991;20:29–36.

19. Valerdi JJ, Tejedor M, Illarramendi JJ, et al. Neoadjuvant chemotherapy and radiotherapy in locally advanced esophagus carcinoma: long-term results. Int J Radiat Oncol Biol Phys 1993;27:843–7.

20. Berger AC, Farma J, Scott WJ, et al. Complete response to neoadjuvant chemoradiotherapy in esophageal carcinoma is associated with significantly improved survival. J Clin Oncol 2005;23:4330–7.

21. Makary MA, Kiernan PD, Sheridan MJ, et al. Multimodality treatment for esophageal cancer: the role of surgery and neoadjuvant therapy. Am Surg 2003;69: 693–700.

22. Stahl M, Stuschke M, Lehmann N, et al. Chemoradiation with and without surgery in patients with locally advanced squamous cell carcinoma of the esophagus. J Clin Oncol 2005;23:2310–7.

23. Heath EI, Burtness BA, Heitmiller RF, et al. Phase II evaluation of preoperative chemoradiation and postoperative adjuvant chemotherapy for squamous cell and adenocarcinoma of the esophagus. J Clin Oncol 2000;18:868–76.

24. Forastiere AA, Orringer MB, Perez-Tamayo C, et al. Preoperative chemoradiation followed by transhiatal esophagectomy for carcinoma of the esophagus: final report. J Clin Oncol 1993;11:1118–23.

25. Geh JI. The use of chemoradiotherapy in oesophageal cancer. Eur J Cancer 2002;38:300–13.
26. Herskovic A, Martz K, al-Sarraf M, et al. Combined chemotherapy and radiotherapy compared with radiotherapy alone in patients with cancer of the esophagus. N Engl J Med 1992;326:1593–8.
27. Cooper JS, Guo MD, Herskovic A, et al. Chemoradiotherapy of locally advanced esophageal cancer: long-term follow-up of a prospective randomized trial (RTOG 85-01). Radiation Therapy Oncology Group. JAMA 1999;281:1623–7.
28. Minsky BD, Pajak TF, Ginsberg RJ, et al. INT 0123 (Radiation Therapy Oncology Group 94-05) phase III trial of combined-modality therapy for esophageal cancer: high-dose versus standard-dose radiation therapy. J Clin Oncol 2002;20:1167–74.
29. Gaspar LE, Winter K, Kocha WI, et al. A phase I/II study of external beam radiation, brachytherapy, and concurrent chemotherapy for patients with localized carcinoma of the esophagus (Radiation Therapy Oncology Group Study 9207): final report. Cancer 2000;88:988–95.
30. Bosset JF, Gignoux M, Triboulet JP, et al. Chemoradiotherapy followed by surgery compared with surgery alone in squamous-cell cancer of the esophagus. N Engl J Med 1997;337:161–7.
31. Urba SG, Orringer MB, Turrisi A, et al. Randomized trial of preoperative chemoradiation versus surgery alone in patients with locoregional esophageal carcinoma. J Clin Oncol 2001;19:305–13.
32. Walsh TN, Noonan N, Hollywood D, et al. A comparison of multimodal therapy and surgery for esophageal adenocarcinoma. N Engl J Med 1996; 335:462–7.
33. Orringer MB, Marshall B, Iannettoni MD. Transhiatal esophagectomy: clinical experience and refinements. Ann Surg 1999;230:392–400.
34. Burmeister BH, Smithers BM, Gebski V, et al. Surgery alone versus chemoradiotherapy followed by surgery for resectable cancer of the oesophagus: a randomised controlled phase III trial. Lancet Oncol 2005;6:659–68.
35. Tepper J, Krasna MJ, Niedzwiecki D, et al. Phase III trial of trimodality therapy with cisplatin, fluorouracil, radiotherapy, and surgery compared with surgery alone for esophageal cancer: CALGB 9781. J Clin Oncol 2008;26:1086–92.
36. Stahl M, Wilke H, Lehmann N, et al. GOCS. Long-term results of a phase III study investigating chemoradiation with and without surgery in locally advanced squamous cell carcinoma (LA-SCC) of the esophagus [abstract 4530]. In Proceedings of American Society of Clinical Oncology Annual Meeting. Chicago: 2008.
37. Bedenne L, Michel P, Bouche O, et al. Chemoradiation followed by surgery compared with chemoradiation alone in squamous cancer of the esophagus: FFCD 9102. J Clin Oncol 2007;25:1160–8.
38. Carstens H, Albertsson M, Friesland S, et al. A randomized trial of chemoradiotherapy versus surgery alone in patients with resectable esophageal cancer [abstract 4530]. American Society of Clinical Oncology 2007.
39. Adelstein DJ, Rice TW, Rybicki LA, et al. Does paclitaxel improve the chemoradiotherapy of locoregionally advanced esophageal cancer? A nonrandomized comparison with fluorouracil-based therapy. J Clin Oncol 2000;18: 2032–9.
40. Blanke CD, Choy H, Teng M, et al. Concurrent paclitaxel and thoracic irradiation for locally advanced esophageal cancer. Semin Radiat Oncol 1999;9:43–52.

41. Urba SG, Orringer MB, Ianettonni M, et al. Concurrent cisplatin, paclitaxel, and radiotherapy as preoperative treatment for patients with locoregional esophageal carcinoma. Cancer 2003;98:2177–83.
42. Brenner B, Ilson DH, Minsky BD, et al. Phase I trial of combined-modality therapy for localized esophageal cancer: escalating doses of continuous-infusion paclitaxel with cisplatin and concurrent radiation therapy. J Clin Oncol 2004;22:45–52.
43. Safran H, Gaissert H, Akerman P, et al. Paclitaxel, cisplatin, and concurrent radiation for esophageal cancer. Cancer Invest 2001;19:1–7.
44. van Meerten E, Muller K, Tilanus HW, et al. Neoadjuvant concurrent chemoradiation with weekly paclitaxel and carboplatin for patients with oesophageal cancer: a phase II study. Br J Cancer 2006;94:1389–94.
45. Henry LR, Goldberg M, Scott W, et al. Induction cisplatin and paclitaxel followed by combination chemoradiotherapy with 5-fluorouracil, cisplatin, and paclitaxel before resection in localized esophageal cancer: a phase II report. Ann Surg Oncol 2006;13:214–20.
46. Meluch AA, Greco FA, Gray JR, et al. Preoperative therapy with concurrent paclitaxel/carboplatin/infusional 5-FU and radiation therapy in locoregional esophageal cancer: final results of a Minnie Pearl Cancer Research Network phase II trial. Cancer J 2003;9:251–60.
47. Weiner LM, Colarusso P, Goldberg M, et al. Combined-modality therapy for esophageal cancer: phase I trial of escalating doses of paclitaxel in combination with cisplatin, 5-fluorouracil, and high-dose radiation before esophagectomy. Semin Oncol 1997;24:S19–95.
48. Wright CD, Wain JC, Lynch TJ, et al. Induction therapy for esophageal cancer with paclitaxel and hyperfractionated radiotherapy: a phase I and II study. J Thorac Cardiovasc Surg 1997;114:811–5.
49. Roof KS, Coen J, Lynch TJ, et al. Concurrent cisplatin, 5-FU, paclitaxel, and radiation therapy in patients with locally advanced esophageal cancer. Int J Radiat Oncol Biol Phys 2006;65:1120–8.
50. Ilson DH, Saltz L, Enzinger P, et al. Phase II trial of weekly irinotecan plus cisplatin in advanced esophageal cancer. J Clin Oncol 1999;17:3270–5.
51. Enzinger P, Mamon H, Choi N, et al. Phase II cisplatin, irinotecan, celecoxib and concurrent radiation therapy followed by surgery for locally advanced esophageal cancer [abstract 35]. Proceedings of the Gastrointestinals American Society of Clinical Oncologists 2004.
52. Ilson DH, Bains M, Kelsen DP, et al. Phase I trial of escalating-dose irinotecan given weekly with cisplatin and concurrent radiotherapy in locally advanced esophageal cancer. J Clin Oncol 2003;21:2926–32.
53. Ku G, Bains M, Rizk N, et al. Phase II trial of pre-operative cisplatin/irinotecan and radiotherapy for locally advanced esophageal cancer: PET scan after induction therapy may identify early treatment failure [abstract 9]. Proceedings of the Gastrointestinals American Society of Clinical Oncologists 2007.
54. Ajani JA, Winter K, Komaki R, et al. Phase II randomized trial of two nonoperative regimens of induction chemotherapy followed by chemoradiation in patients with localized carcinoma of the esophagus: RTOG 0113. J Clin Oncol 2008;26(28):4551–6.
55. Downey RJ, Akhurst T, Ilson D, et al. Whole body [18]FDG-PET and the response of esophageal cancer to induction therapy: results of a prospective trial. J Clin Oncol 2003;21:428–32.

56. Flamen P, Van Cutsem E, Lerut A, et al. Positron emission tomography for assessment of the response to induction radiochemotherapy in locally advanced oesophageal cancer. Ann Oncol 2002;13:361–8.

57. Ott K, Weber WA, Lordick F, et al. Metabolic imaging predicts response, survival, and recurrence in adenocarcinomas of the esophagogastric junction. J Clin Oncol 2006;24:4692–8.

58. Weber WA, Ott K, Becker K, et al. Prediction of response to preoperative chemotherapy in adenocarcinomas of the esophagogastric junction by metabolic imaging. J Clin Oncol 2001;19:3058–85.

59. Lordick F, Ott K, Krause BJ, et al. PET to assess early metabolic response and to guide treatment of adenocarcinoma of the oesophagogastric junction: the MUNICON phase II trial. Lancet Oncol 2007;8:797–805.

60. Lordick F, Ott K, Krause B, et al. Salvage radiochemotherapy in locally advanced gastroesophageal junction tumors that are metabolically resistant to induction chemotherapy: the MUNICON-2 trial [abstract 104]. Proceedings of the Gastrointestinals American Society of Clinical Oncologists 2008.

Surgical Palliation for Barrett's Esophagus Cancer

Irfan Qureshi, MD[a],*, Manisha Shende, MD[b], James D. Luketich, MD[c]

KEYWORDS

- Barrett's esophagus • Gastroesophageal reflux
- Esophageal adenocarcinoma • Palliation
- Stent • Radiotherapy • Brachytherapy

Esophageal adenocarcinoma was first described by White in 1898. At that time, it was believed that this malignancy was an extension of gastric tumors.[1,2] In 1950, Norman Barrett[3] published his treatise on the columnar-lined segment of tissue located in the distal esophagus. He also noted the development of adenocarcinoma in this area. Various reports followed that described the development of adenocarcinoma from this specialized epithelium. Over the next 50 years, the association between gastroesophageal reflux, Barrett's esophagus, and adenocarcinoma became well established.

Clinical studies have linked the development of adenocarcinoma to the presence of chronic gastroesophageal reflux and Barrett's esophagus. In 1999, Lagergren and colleagues[4] found in a case-control study that subjects who had standing reflux symptoms were 43 times more likely to develop adenocarcinoma as compared with asymptomatic individuals. Among subjects with chronic reflux, it has also been shown that Barrett's esophagus is a major indicator for cancer. In 2004, Solaymani-Dodaran and colleagues[5] found that subjects who have Barrett's esophagus have a 30 times higher risk of adenocarcinoma compared with subjects who have reflux but no Barrett's. Whereas subjects who have Barrett's esophagus have a 50 to 100 fold increased risk of esophageal cancer as compared with the general population,[6] subjects who have reflux and no Barrett's have only a 3.1 times increased risk as compared with the general population. In addition, a greater increase in the development of carcinoma is seen with the progression of Barrett's esophagus to dysplasia.[7,8]

[a] Heart, Lung and Esophageal Surgery Institute, University of Pittsburgh Medical Center, Kaufmann Building Suite 401, 3471 Fifth Avenue, Pittsburgh, PA, USA
[b] Heart, Lung and Esophageal Surgery Institute, University of Pittsburgh Medical Center, 200 Lothrop Street, Suite C-700, Presbyterian University Hospital, Pittsburgh, PA, USA
[c] Heart, Lung and Esophageal Surgery Institute, University of Pittsburgh Medical Center, 200 Lothrop Street, Suite C-800, Presbyterian University Hospital, Pittsburgh, PA, USA
* Corresponding author.
E-mail address: qureshiir@upmc.edu (I. Qureshi).

Surg Oncol Clin N Am 18 (2009) 547–560
doi:10.1016/j.soc.2009.03.009
1055-3207/09/$ – see front matter © 2009 Elsevier Inc. All rights reserved.

surgonc.theclinics.com

Repeated mucosal injury in the setting of acid reflux exposure causes squamous epithelium metaplasia to columnar epithelium containing goblet cells. Over time, the transition from Barrett's epithelium to adenocarcinoma progresses through a meta-plasia–dysplasia–carcinoma sequence, as seen in many patients.[9] Therefore, the presence of Barrett's is considered a premalignant condition and carries an increased risk of cancer.[6] It is estimated that patients with Barrett's esophagus have a risk of 0.5% per year of developing adenocarcinoma.[10] Risk factors for the development of Barrett's esophagus include male sex, obesity, age greater than 50 years, smoking history, and greater than 5-year history of reflux symptoms.[11]

Adenocarcinoma of the esophagus was previously rarer than esophageal squa-mous cell carcinoma. However, with increasing rates of gastroesophageal reflux and chronic tissue injury, esophageal adenocarcinoma has exhibited the fastest increasing incidence of any malignancy in the United States, with yearly increases in incidence exceeding 20% since 1975.[12–14] Demographically, the bulk of this increase has occurred in white men, who now have an average incidence as high as 5.3 per 100,000.[15,16] White women and black men have also begun to show higher incidences.[17] Consequently, adenocarcinoma has replaced squamous cell carcinoma as the most common malignancy of the esophagus.[18] Advanced esophageal cancer carries an overall poor prognosis. Most patients diagnosed with esophageal malignancy will have incurable disease and require palliative therapy.

ADENOCARCINOMA OF THE ESOPHAGUS AND GASTROESOPHAGEAL JUNCTION

The distinction between esophageal and gastric tumors is difficult to ascertain in path-ological specimens and the exact etiology of the carcinoma continues to be a difficult task. Tumors in the esophagus may migrate distally, whereas proximal extension may be seen in GEJ tumors. For this reason, assigning an exact etiology to some tumors can be confusing. A classification system for adenocarcinoma of the esophagus and GEJ tumors was created by Siewert and colleagues.[19] In this classification system, the tumors are divided into types according to the location of the tumor center. Barrett's adenocarcinomas of the distal esophagus are classified as type 1 tumors. Type 2 tumors are centered at the GEJ and Type 3 are subcardial gastric tumors. Pathophysio-logically, GEJ tumors and esophageal adenocarcinomas share similar features.[20] Both cancers also share similar risk factors with increased incidence of both in patients with long term gastroesophageal reflux. Studies have also shown that survival and lymph node involvement in both cancers are similar.[21] Therefore, GEJ tumors and esophageal adenocarcinomas are evaluated and treated similarly.

Etiology and Pathophysiology

The specific factors responsible for the prevalence of esophageal adenocarcinomas are unknown. However, chronic acid and bile reflux exposure plays a key role in the development of Barrett's metaplasia.[22] Chronic distal esophageal acid inflammation leads to a variety of cellular changes, including low mucosal glutaminase levels, altered levels of mucosal protein synthesis, and loss of disaccharidase activity.[23] In addition, a variety of intracellular pathways are altered by reflux in the setting of Bar-rett's metaplasia, including MAP kinase activation[24] and up-regulation of COX-2 expression.[25] Bile acids also play a role in carcinogenesis by inducing mitochondrial and cell membrane damage.

The pathogenesis of esophageal and GEJ cancer includes the accumulation of multiple genetic alterations over time. The loss of heterozygosity of tumor-suppressor genes, such as p53, the adenomatous polyposis coli (APC) gene, the gene deleted in colorectal cancer (DCC) and MTS1 (p16), is correlated with progression from metaplasia to dysplasia and finally to carcinoma.[26] However, the current data on these genetic alterations is not sufficient to allow routine testing of these markers in clinical practice.

Incidence and Prognosis

Cancers of the esophagus and GEJ are diagnosed in more than 400,000 patients per year worldwide, making them the eighth most common malignancy and sixth on the list of cancer mortality causes.[27] The true incidence is difficult to ascertain since cancers of the GEJ are sometimes classified as gastric cancer and other times as esophageal cancer. However, both cancers have treatment options that are similar.

Cancer of the esophagus carries a poor prognosis with a 5-year survival rate of less than 20%.[28] More than two-thirds of the esophageal cancers diagnosed in Western countries are adenocarcinomas. Of the patients diagnosed with cancer of the esophagus and GEJ, more than 50% will have incurable disease due to metastases or a poor medical condition and will present with dysphagia or associated problems, such as tracheoesophageal fistula.[29]

Treatment

Treatment options for patients with advanced esophageal tumors include a wide variety of currently available palliative techniques. Most patients with incurable esophageal cancer live no longer than 6 months from the time of diagnosis. The aim of most treatments is to maintain oral food intake and to avoid serious complications. Critical factors that influence the plan for therapy should include the tumor stage, the overall health of the patient, and the goal of the therapy. The palliative treatments available can be divided into endoscopic therapies, including esophageal stent therapy, and nonendoscopic procedures, such as radiotherapy and brachytherapy (**Table 1**).[30]

Stents
Currently the most widely used palliative method is the placement of a self-expanding esophageal stent to relieve malignant dysphagia.[31] The use of stents for the palliation

Table 1	
Palliative modalities for esophageal carcinoma	
Modality	
Endoscopic techniques	Stent placement
	Laser therapy:
	Thermal (Nd:YAG)
	Photodynamic therapy
	Dilation
	Electrocoagulation (BICAP probe)
	Chemical injection therapy
	Nutritional support
	Nasoenteric feeding tube
	Percutaneous endoscopic gastrostomy (PEG)
Non-endoscopic techniques	Surgery
	Radiation therapy:
	External-beam radiotherapy
	Intraluminal radiotherapy (brachytherapy)
	Chemotherapy

From Siersema PD. New developments in palliative therapy. Best Pract Res Clin Gastroenterol 2006;20:959–78; with permission.

of incurable esophageal adenocarcinoma has been studied extensively since 1990.[32,33] All stents aim to ensure passage of a normal diet. They should expand in a nontraumatic fashion when placed and resist migration but allow repositioning or removal. However, no modern stent can achieve all these goals.

Placement of an esophageal stent can be preformed in an outpatient or inpatient setting. Many patients present with moderate-to-severe dysphagia and varying degrees of dehydration and malnutrition. In this setting, it has been advantageous for the patient and the family to consider immediate stenting. The technical success rate of placement approaches 100%; however, severe pain during placement, failure of the stent to release from the introduction system, and immediate stent migration due to distal placement can limit success. The dysphagia score improves rapidly after placement. Most patients initially present with a dysphagia score of 3 (able to consume only liquids) and improve to a dysphagia score of 1 (eating most solid foods) immediately after the placement of an esophageal stent. Even though stents have the unique ability to provide palliation of malignant dysphagia, the use of these stents is sometimes associated with complications, which include esophageal perforation, aspiration pneumonia, fever, bleeding from a traumatic placement, and severe retrosternal pain. Approximately 5%–15% of patients who have stents placed present with such complications. A common long-term problem in these patients is recurrent dysphagia. The most common reasons for recurrent dysphagia in stent therapy are migration of the stent and malignant and benign tumor overgrowth into the stent.[34] Approximately 30%–45% of patients treated with stents have recurrent symptoms of dysphagia. In our study of over 100 stents placed in 100 subjects for malignant dysphagia, 85% of the subjects had immediate relief from dysphagia. Of these subjects, 49% had palliation of their symptoms until death (mean interval 125 days). The other 51% required reintervention at a mean interval of 82 days. Tumor overgrowth/ingrowth was the most frequent reason for intervention.[35]

Types of stents The first-generation metallic stents were uncovered, which allowed tumor ingrowth. Newer stents are covered or partially covered.[36] **Table 2** shows the characteristics of the various stents used for palliative treatment.[30]

The Wallstent (Boston Scientific, Natick, Massachusetts) is a cobalt-based alloy stent that is formed into a tubular mesh and is currently available in two separate designs: the Wallstent II (available in the United States) and the Flamingo Wallstent (available only in Europe) (**Fig. 1**).[30] The Wallstent II has a diameter of 20 mm at the midsection and flares to 28 mm at both ends. The stent is covered with a silicone polymer layer and can be repositioned during placement. The Flamingo Wallstent is placed mainly in the distal esophagus and gastric cardiac region. It is covered with a polyurethane layer that extends to within 2 cm of each end of the stent. The conical shape of this stent is designed for specific esophageal accommodation and is manufactured to apply variable radial forces throughout the length of the stent to specifically contour to the shape of the esophagus and prevent migration. After placement of the Wallstent, shortening of approximately 20%–30% occurs.[30] The Flamingo Wallstent is available in a large diameter version (30 mm proximal diameter; 20 mm distal diameter and a small diameter model, 24 mm proximal diameter; 16 mm distal diameter).

The Z-Stent (Wilson-Cook Medical, Winston-Salem, North Carolina) is a stent that consists of a woven wire mesh of stainless steel completely covered by polyethylene. The stent has an introduction system that is more complex than other metallic stents. The dimensions of this stent include a midsection diameter of either 18 mm or 22 mm with both ends flaring to 25 mm. The Z-Stent has the advantage of not shortening upon insertion; however, it is the least flexible of all metallic stents currently available.

Table 2
Characteristics of currently available stents

Stent Type	Covering	Length (cm)	Diameter (mm)	Release System	Radial Force	Degree of Shortening	Flexibility	Stent Material	Manufacturer
Ultraflex	Partial	10,12,15	18,22	Proximal/distal	Low	30%–40%	High	Nitinol	Boston Scientific, Natick, Mass.
Wallstent II	Partial	10,15	20	Distal	High	20%–30%	Moderate	Cobalt-based alloy	Boston Scientific, Natick, Mass.
Flamingo Wallstent	Partial	12 / 14	Prox:24/dist:16 Prox:30/dist:20	Distal	High	20%–30%	Moderate	Cobalt-based alloy	Boston Scientific, Natick, Mass.
Z-stent	Full	6,8,10,12,14	18,22	Distal	Moderate	None	Low	Stainless steel	Wilson-Cook Medical, Winston-Salem, North Carolina
Choo stent	Full	8,11,14,17	18	Distal	Moderate	None	Low	Nitinol	MI Tech, Seoul, Korea

From Siersema PD. New developments in palliative therapy. Best Pract Res Clin Gastroenterol 2006;20:959–78; with permission.

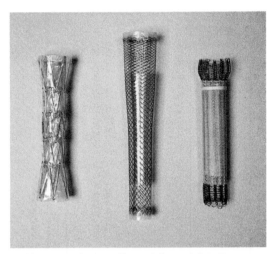

Fig. 1. Currently available covered stents (from *left* to *right*): European version of Z-stent, Flamingo Wallstent, and Ultraflex stent. *From* Siersema PD: New developments in palliative therapy. Best Pract Res Clin Gastroenterol 2006;20:959–78; with permission.

The Ultraflex stent (Boston Scientific) is a metallic stent that has a knitted nitinol wire tube; the covered version of this stent has a polyurethane layer that occupies the midsection of the stent extending to within 1.5 cm of either end. Upon insertion of this stent, a shortening of 30%–40% is observed. The Ultraflex stent exerts the least radial force of all the metallic stents.

Studies involving metallic stents In 1996, May and colleagues[37] performed a retrospective study in 96 subjects, analyzing all of the metallic stents available at that time. They reported no difference in the rate of complications associated with the different metallic stents. In 2001, the results of a study comparing three metallic stents (the Z-Stent, Flamingo Wallstent and Ultraflex stent) were published. In this prospective trial of 100 subjects randomized to one of the three stents, Siersema and colleagues[38] found no significant difference in dysphagia improvement among the different stents, and similar complication rates among the three types of stents.

Gastroesophageal junction stents Adenocarcinoma of the GEJ has presented a difficult situation in terms of palliative treatment. Stents placed for palliative purposes at the GEJ have been associated with many complications.[39] Some of these complications are similar to the ones experienced by patients with esophageal stents. However, GEJ stents experience higher distal migration rates than similar stents placed in a more proximal location. GEJ-placed stents also increase the frequency of bleeding and, more important, have been reported to result in an inferior quality of swallowing after placement compared with stents placed in a more proximal location. In our study of 100 subjects treated for malignant dysphagia with expandable metal stents, described above, a majority (58 subjects) had tumors at the GEJ. We saw an 8% migration rate and 11% of the subjects had severe recalcitrant reflux despite lifestyle changes and proton-pump inhibitor (PPI) administration.[35]

A major complication attributed to the placement of GEJ stents is the severity of reflux symptoms that the patients experience. To minimize this reflux, a family of metal stents has been designed with the cover of the stent extending beyond the lower metal cage to form a windsock-type antireflux valve.[29] In a 2001 study, Dua and colleagues[40] studied the Z-Stent with the antireflux valve in 11 subjects. This stent was effective in preventing reflux symptoms. In a separate study, the effectiveness of a modified antireflux stent was compared with a nonmodified Flamingo Wallstent. In this study, 25 subjects were randomized to the antireflux stent and 25 were randomized to a Wallstent. Three of the 25 subjects (12%) who had the antireflux stent showed symptoms of reflux compared with 24 of the 25 (96%) subjects who had a nonmodified Wallstent (*P*<.001). No differences in dysphagia improvement, complication rates, or reintervention rates were seen.[41]

Not all studies, however, have shown promising results using the modified antireflux stents. In 2004, Homs and colleagues[42] compared the FerX-Ella (Ella-CS, Hradec Kralove, Czech Republic) stent with an antireflux valve with an open version of the stent in a randomized study. After 24-hr pH monitoring, they found increased esophageal acid exposure in subjects who received an antireflux version of the stent. One possible explanation for this finding could be the design of the stent used in the study. Clearly, the appropriate stent and stent placement for GEJ tumors needs further evaluation and research. PPIs can be used in combination with stents to alleviate reflux symptoms in patients who have GEJ tumors. This medical therapy can be an adjunctive treatment in both patients who have modified antireflux stents and patients who have nonmodified stents. Many institutions implement this strategy to limit the level of discomfort that is present in these incurable patients.

Alterations in stent design New stent designs have been created to limit the complications that are seen with stent placement, such as migration and benign and malignant tissue overgrowth.. These include the Polyflex and Niti-S stents.

The Polyflex stent (Rusch AG, Kernen, Germany) is a newly designed self-expandable stent that is made of plastic and silicone rather than metal (**Fig. 2**).[30] It is completely covered and flares to 25 mm at the proximal end. In 2003, Dormann and colleagues[43] published a prospective cohort study analyzing the Polyflex stent in 33 subjects with malignant dysphagia. After a mean follow-up of 150 days, no stent occlusion due to benign tissue overgrowth was seen. In this study, migration of the Polyflex stent was seen in only 6% of the study group. However, the study did find that 10% of subjects had stent occlusion due malignant tumor overgrowth. In contrast, migration was a major complication in our experience with the Polyflex stent.

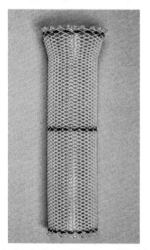

Fig. 2. Polyflex silicone-covered stent. *From* Siersema PD: New developments in palliative therapy. Best Pract Res Clin Gastroenterol 2006;20:959–78; with permission.

We placed 58 Polyflex stents in 38 subjects who had a variety of conditions, including malignant and benign esophageal strictures, leaks, and tracheoesophageal fistulas. Although dysphagia improved significantly following stent placement, migration occurred in 73% of the subjects (63% of placed stents). Mean interval to reintervention was 46 days and migration was the major factor underlying the need for reintervention.[44] Other investigators have reported variable rates of migration from 20%–57%.[45–47] Clearly, further exploration is needed to delineate both optimal placement and candidate for the Polyflex stent.

The second newly designed stent is the Niti-S stent (Taewong Medical, Seoul, Korea). Its unique design, with an inner polyurethane layer and outer, uncovered, nitinol wire tubes, allows the stent to embed deep within the esophagus, thereby limiting the rate of migration. In a study published in 2006, Verschuur and colleagues[48] prospectively treated 42 subjects with the Niti-S stent, with promising results: distal migration was observed in only 7%; tumor and nontumor overgrowth was found in only 5%. The mean follow-up was 6 months.

Many studies have examined covered and uncovered metallic stents, as well as the Polyflex and Niti-S stents. The completely covered stents have shown superior results in preventing tissue overgrowth. In a recent study comparing the outcomes of 125 subjects randomized to either the Ultraflex stent (a partially covered metal stent), the Polyflex stent, or the Niti-S stent, migration was seen most frequently with the Polyflex stent. Tumor ingrowth and overgrowth occurred most frequently with the Ultraflex stent, and relief from dysphagia was the same for all three stents.[49] Further randomized, prospective studies comparing completely covered stents with uncovered or partially covered stents are needed before a definitive conclusion can be reached as to the most appropriate stent for effective palliative treatment of patients with esophageal adenocarcinoma.

Stents for fistulas Another complication that can arise in a patient who has an advanced esophageal tumor is the development of a fistula. Contact between the tumor in the esophagus and surrounding tissue, such as the trachea and the aorta, can lead to the development of a fistula from the esophagus to the surrounding structures. Fistulas can also form after radiation or laser treatment that causes radiation esophagitis. Because of the advanced stage of the tumor and the incurable nature of the disease, aggressive surgical options are not appropriate for maintaining quality of life. Surgical therapy is associated with a mortality rate of 50% in such patients. Therefore, the best therapy for the closure of fistula is often an appropriately sized, covered, esophageal stent. Complete closure of the fistula can be established in more than 90% of patients with similar results using different stents.[50,51]

Laser therapy
Neodymium yttrium–aluminum–garnet (Nd:YAG) laser is another treatment option for palliation of malignant dysphagia. The treatment is most effective for lesions that are exophytic, less than 6 cm in diameter, and located in the midesophagus. Treatment of circumferential tumors with YAG laser causes stricture formation. A significant improvement in dysphagia after YAG treatment occurs in 35%–80% of patients.[52,53] Multiple treatments are required to achieve palliation, therefore requiring reassessment at 4–6 week intervals. In 5%–10% of patients, perforation and fistula formation is seen in the esophagus following YAG treatment.

Photodynamic therapy
Photodynamic therapy (PDT) uses endoscopically administered light of a specific wavelength to activate a previously administered photosensitizer in malignant tissue.

Activation of the photosensitizer leads to an oxidative photochemical reaction that results in mucosal destruction. Porfimer sodium (Photofrin) has been the most commonly used photosensitizer. Tumor response is seen after two treatments. Skin photosensitivity is a frequent complication and necessitates 4–6 weeks of sunlight avoidance. Other complications associated with PDT include perforation, fistula formation, and strictures in 30% of patients. PDT is an expensive option because of the high costs of the light source and photosensitizer and because the treatment must be repeated every 8 weeks.

We investigated PDT palliation of malignant dysphagia in a study of 215 esophageal cancer subjects, the largest published to date. In 15% of these patients, PDT was administered to relieve dysphagia resulting from tumor ingrowth or overgrowth in a previously placed stent. The treatment was effective 85% of the time. Following PDT, mean dysphagia score improved and the mean dysphagia-free interval was 66 days. Sunburn was the most frequent complication, occurring in 6% of the patients.[54]

Lightdale and colleagues[55] compared PDT with the YAG laser. PDT resulted in similar improvements in dysphagia score and had similar complication rates but greater side effects than the YAG laser. However, in a separate study, PDT improved performance status and gave a longer duration of response as compared with the YAG laser.[56] Because PDT has greater side effects, higher costs, and requires repeated treatments, it is more effective if combined with other palliative treatment modalities.

Brachytherapy

Inoperable esophageal adenocarcinoma was once treated with external beam radiation therapy to the area with the tumor. This was followed by intraluminal radiotherapy (brachytherapy) 2–3 weeks after completion of external beam radiotherapy. However, brachytherapy has become a stand-alone option for palliative treatment. Brachytherapy focuses a maximum dose of radiation directly to the tumor without damaging surrounding normal tissue, an advantage lacking in external beam radiotherapy.

To administer this localized radiation treatment, a flexible applicator is passed into the esophagus over a guidewire. Iridium (Ir^{192}) is then used as the radiation source for the treatment. Various rates of therapy can be administered with a low-dose delivery of 0.4–2 Gy per hour, a medium dose of 2–12 Gy per hour, and a high dose of 12 or more Gy per hour. Palliation of dysphagia is best achieved with 7.5 to 20 Gy administered in 1 to 3 fractions.[57,58] Studies of brachytherapy for treatment of patients with dysphagia have also used treatment schedules with a single dose of 12–15 Gy.[59,60] A 1998 study by Sur and colleagues[57] compared various doses of brachytherapy in 172 subjects who were randomized to receive 12 Gy in 2 fractions, 16 Gy in 2 fractions, or 18 Gy in 3 fractions. The study showed that subjects who received 16 Gy in 2 fractions or 18 Gy in 3 fractions had better dysphagia-free survival than the subjects who received 12 Gy in 2 fractions. Additionally, smaller tumor growth was seen in the subjects receiving 16 or 18 Gy than in subjects receiving 12 Gy treatments.

Brachytherapy is a safe treatment option for palliation of malignant dysphagia. Complication rates are reported to be low and consist of mild retrosternal pain, fistula formation, and radiation esophagitis. Persistence of the tumor, tumor recurrence, and benign stricture formation is seen in 10% to 40% of patients following brachytherapy. Such complications are usually treated with another dose of brachytherapy or placement of a stent.[61]

Brachytherapy treatment has been compared with stent placement and laser therapy for long-term palliation. Homs and colleagues[62] compared 12 Gy, single-dose brachytherapy with the use of Ultraflex stent treatment in 200 randomized subjects. The study found that stent therapy improved dysphagia more rapidly than brachytherapy, but long-term relief was superior with brachytherapy. Fewer complications occurred with brachytherapy treatment as compared with stents (21% versus 33%). Brachytherapy treatment has also been analyzed for treatment of dysphagia in combination with laser therapy. In a prospective, randomized trial, 20 subjects were treated with laser therapy alone and 19 with laser therapy and brachytherapy. In subjects who had squamous cell carcinoma, a prolonged dysphagia-free interval was seen after combination treatment. However, the study showed no difference in dysphagia-free survival in adenocarcinoma subjects, nor in overall survival.[63]

Surgical treatment

The 5-year survival rate for all patients with esophageal cancer remains only 15%–20%, due in part to the advanced stage of disease at presentation. Survival for these patients often is no longer than 6 months. Therefore, surgery remains a poor alternative for this group due to the high morbidity and mortality associated with esophagectomy. Additionally, quality-of-life studies on patients afflicted with esophageal cancer who have undergone esophageal resection have shown that, early in the postoperative phase, most aspects of the patients' quality of life significantly deteriorate.[64] With such a short survival period, the role of palliative resections is becoming less applicable, because other less invasive methods of palliation now exist.

Esophagectomy is still considered the mainstay of treatment for patients who have localized esophageal cancer. The ability to perform an R0 resection with clear resection margins has been consistently shown to have the best prognosis. However, patients who have advanced esophageal cancer with T4 disease or distant metastases have such a poor prognosis that surgery is rarely indicated in these cases. Endoscopic palliative therapies offer patients who are not candidates for surgery the opportunity to relieve their dysphagia, improve their quality of life and, in some cases, resume their everyday activities. Some patients will, however, fail endoscopic palliation with stents or PDT. A very limited number of these patients may be considered for surgical resection or a bypass to relieve dysphagia. We must emphasize that this option should only be offered to patients who have failed endoscopic methods of palliation, are in otherwise reasonable health and have access to a center that offers esophagectomy with low morbidity and mortality. Another indication for a palliative resection may be a patient who presents with severe bleeding from a tumor that fails conventional management with endoscopic epinephrine injection and/or coagulation, PDT, laser fulguration, or, in some cases, of tracheoesophageal fistula. Again, endoscopic therapies should be considered first and caution should be exercised before offering a surgical option.

Quality of Life

The main goal of palliative treatment for incurable esophageal adenocarcinoma and GEJ tumors is for preservation of health-related quality of life. Currently, very few studies evaluate quality of life after palliative treatment for esophageal cancer. The studies that have examined quality of life after treatment show that dysphagia scores improve for a short period of time. However, other aspects defining quality of life decline over long-term follow-up.[29]

SUMMARY

The incidence of adenocarcinoma arising in the setting of Barrett's esophagus is increasing faster than any other malignancy. Esophageal adenocarcinoma has become more prevalent than esophageal squamous cell carcinoma. Advanced stage esophageal adenocarcinoma has a poor prognosis with 50% of patients having incurable disease at diagnosis due to metastases. Determining appropriate treatment options for incurable esophageal adenocarcinoma remains a critical challenge. Patients afflicted with such an aggressive form of cancer usually require palliation of their symptoms rather than aggressive surgical options, such as esophagectomy.

Current treatment options, such as stents, PDT, laser therapy, and brachytherapy all offer short-term relief of dysphagia; however, each therapy continues to have the complication of recurrent dysphagia with the additional complication of recurrent migration associated with the use of stents. None of the currently available treatment options for palliation are optimal in achieving sustained malignant dysphagia relief with minimal morbidity and mortality.

One option that may resolve the complication of long-term dysphagia is the use of multimodality treatment. Using brachytherapy along with stent placement may allow long-term palliation of dysphagia. However, this combination treatment will most likely require multiple hospital visits and longer hospital stays, whereas the current treatment options can be administered in an outpatient setting. The combination of PDT and a metallic stent yields good results in patients with a life expectancy of less than 6 months. Future randomized trials will allow a better understanding of combination therapy as compared with monotherapy for dysphagia relief and improvement of quality of life. Future studies are also needed to determine variations in stent therapy that will be more effective in alleviating symptoms. Drug-eluting stents have been considered in prevention of tumor growth; however, further evaluations are needed to ensure the efficacy of such stents in providing palliative treatment.

ACKNOWLEDGMENTS

We thank Shannon Wyszomierski for editing the manuscript.

REFERENCES

1. Armstrong RA, Blalcock JB, Carrera G. Adenocarcinoma of the middle third of the esophagus arising from ectopic gastric mucosa. J Thorac Surg 1959;37:398–403.
2. Hewlett AW. The superficial glands of the esophagus. J Exp Med 1901;5:319–32.
3. Barrett NR. Chronic peptic ulcer of the oesophagus and 'oesophagitis'. Br J Surg 1950;38:175–82.
4. Lagergren J, Bergstrom R, Lindgren A, et al. Symptomatic gastroesophageal reflux as a risk factor for esophageal adenocarcinoma. N Engl J Med 1999;340:825–31.
5. Solaymani-Dodaran M, Logan RF, West J, et al. Risk of oesophageal cancer in Barrett's oesophagus and gastro-oesophageal reflux. Gut 2004;53:1070–4.
6. Cameron AJ, Lomboy CT, Pera M, et al. Adenocarcinoma of the esophagogastric junction and Barrett's esophagus. Gastroenterology 1995;109:1541–6.
7. Conio M, Cameron AJ, Romero Y, et al. Secular trends in the epidemiology and outcome of Barrett's oesophagus in Olmsted County, Minnesota. Gut 2001;48:304–9.
8. Rudolph RE, Vaughan TL, Storer BE, et al. Effect of segment length on risk for neoplastic progression in patients with Barrett's esophagus. Ann Intern Med 2000;132:612–20.
9. Hameeteman W, Tytgat GN, Houthoff HJ, et al. Barrett's esophagus: development of dysplasia and adenocarcinoma. Gastroenterology 1989;96:1249–56.
10. Shaheen NJ, Crosby MA, Bozymski EM, et al. Is there publication bias in the reporting of cancer risk in Barrett's esophagus? Gastroenterology 2000;119:333–8.

11. Devesa SS, Blot WJ, Fraumeni JF Jr. Changing patterns in the incidence of esophageal and gastric carcinoma in the United States. Cancer 1998;83: 2049–53.

12. Blot WJ, Devesa SS, Kneller RW, et al. Rising incidence of adenocarcinoma of the esophagus and gastric cardia. JAMA 1991;265:1287–9.

13. Kubo A, Corley DA. Marked multi-ethnic variation of esophageal and gastric cardia carcinomas within the United States. Am J Gastroenterol 2004;99:582–8.

14. Pohl H, Welch HG. The role of overdiagnosis and reclassification in the marked increase of esophageal adenocarcinoma incidence. J Natl Cancer Inst 2005; 97:142–6.

15. Bollschweiler E, Wolfgarten E, Gutschow C, et al. Demographic variations in the rising incidence of esophageal adenocarcinoma in white males. Cancer 2001;92: 549–55.

16. el-Serag HB. The epidemic of esophageal adenocarcinoma. Gastroenterol Clin North Am 2002;31:421–40, viii.

17. Kubo A, Corley DA. Marked regional variation in adenocarcinomas of the esophagus and the gastric cardia in the United States. Cancer 2002;95:2096–102.

18. Chen X, Yang CS. Esophageal adenocarcinoma: a review and perspectives on the mechanism of carcinogenesis and chemoprevention. Carcinogenesis 2001; 22:1119–29.

19. Siewert JR, Feith M, Werner M, et al. Adenocarcinoma of the esophagogastric junction: results of surgical therapy based on anatomical/topographic classification in 1,002 consecutive patients. Ann Surg 2000;232:353–61.

20. Dolan K, Sutton R, Walker SJ, et al. New classification of oesophageal and gastric carcinomas derived from changing patterns in epidemiology. Br J Cancer 1999; 80:834–42.

21. Wijnhoven BP, Siersema PD, Hop WC, et al. Adenocarcinomas of the distal oesophagus and gastric cardia are one clinical entity. Rotterdam Oesophageal Tumour Study Group. Br J Surg 1999;86:529–35.

22. Theisen J, Peters JH, Stein HJ. Experimental evidence for mutagenic potential of duodenogastric juice on Barrett's esophagus. World J Surg 2003;27:1018–20.

23. Peters JH, DeMeester TR. Esophagus: anatomy physiology and gastroesophageal reflux disease. In: Greenfield LJM, Mulholland M, Oldham KT, editors. Surgery: scientific principles and practice. 3rd edition. Philadelphia: Lippincott, Williams and Wilkins; 2001. p. 671–5.

24. Souza RF, Shewmake K, Pearson S, et al. Acid increases proliferation via ERK and p38 MAPK-mediated increases in cyclooxygenase-2 in Barrett's adenocarcinoma cells. Am J Physiol Gastrointest Liver Physiol 2004;287:G743–8.

25. Hamoui N, Peters JH, Schneider S, et al. Increased acid exposure in patients with gastroesophageal reflux disease influences cyclooxygenase-2 gene expression in the squamous epithelium of the lower esophagus. Arch Surg 2004;139: 712–6 [discussion: 6–7].

26. Raja S, Finkelstein SD, Baksh FK, et al. Correlation between dysplasia and mutations of six tumor suppressor genes in Barrett's esophagus. Ann Thorac Surg 2001;72:1130–5.

27. Parkin DM, Bray FI, Devesa SS. Cancer burden in the year 2000. The global picture. Eur J Cancer 2001;37(Suppl 8):S4–66.

28. Pisani P, Parkin DM, Bray F, et al. Estimates of the worldwide mortality from 25 cancers in 1990. Int J Cancer 1999;83:18–29.

29. Homs MY, Kuipers EJ, Siersema PD. Palliative therapy. J Surg Oncol 2005;92: 246–56.

30. Siersema PD. New developments in palliative therapy. Best Pract Res Clin Gastroenterol 2006;20:959–78.

31. Bartelsman JF, Bruno MJ, Jensema AJ, et al. Palliation of patients with esophago-gastric neoplasms by insertion of a covered expandable modified Gianturco-Z endoprosthesis: experiences in 153 patients. Gastrointest Endosc 2000;51: 134–8.

32. Baron TH. Expandable metal stents for the treatment of cancerous obstruction of the gastrointestinal tract. N Engl J Med 2001;344:1681–7.

33. Ell C, May A. Self-expanding metal stents for palliation of stenosing tumors of the esophagus and cardia: a critical review. Endoscopy 1997;29:392–8.

34. Vakil N, Morris AI, Marcon N, et al. A prospective, randomized, controlled trial of covered expandable metal stents in the palliation of malignant esophageal obstruction at the gastroesophageal junction. Am J Gastroenterol 2001;96: 1791–6.

35. Christie NA, Buenaventura PO, Fernando HC, et al. Results of expandable metal stents for malignant esophageal obstruction in 100 patients: short-term and long-term follow-up. Ann Thorac Surg 2001;71:1797–801 [discussion: 801–2].

36. Homs MY, Steyerberg EW, Kuipers EJ, et al. Causes and treatment of recurrent dysphagia after self-expanding metal stent placement for palliation of esopha-geal carcinoma. Endoscopy 2004;36:880–6.

37. May A, Hahn EG, Ell C. Self-expanding metal stents for palliation of malignant obstruction in the upper gastrointestinal tract. Comparative assessment of three stent types implemented in 96 implantations. J Clin Gastroenterol 1996;22:261–6.

38. Siersema PD, Hop WC, van Blankenstein M, et al. A comparison of 3 types of covered metal stents for the palliation of patients with dysphagia caused by esophagogastric carcinoma: a prospective, randomized study. Gastrointest Endosc 2001;54:145–53.

39. Botterweck AA, Schouten LJ, Volovics A, et al. Trends in incidence of adenocar-cinoma of the oesophagus and gastric cardia in ten European countries. Int J Epidemiol 2000;29:645–54.

40. Dua KS, Kozarek R, Kim J, et al. Self-expanding metal esophageal stent with anti-reflux mechanism. Gastrointest Endosc 2001;53:603–13.

41. Laasch HU, Marriott A, Wilbraham L, et al. Effectiveness of open versus antireflux stents for palliation of distal esophageal carcinoma and prevention of symptom-atic gastroesophageal reflux. Radiology 2002;225:359–65.

42. Homs MY, Wahab PJ, Kuipers EJ, et al. Esophageal stents with antireflux valve for tumors of the distal esophagus and gastric cardia: a randomized trial. Gastroint-est Endosc 2004;60:695–702.

43. Dormann AJ, Eisendrath P, Wigginghaus B, et al. Palliation of esophageal carci-noma with a new self-expanding plastic stent. Endoscopy 2003;35:207–11.

44. Pennathur A, Chang AC, McGrath KM, et al. Polyflex expandable stents in the treatment of esophageal disease: initial experience. Ann Thorac Surg 2008;85: 1968–72 [discussion: 73].

45. Conigliaro R, Battaglia G, Repici A, et al. Polyflex stents for malignant oesopha-geal and oesophagogastric stricture: a prospective, multicentric study. Eur J Gastroenterol Hepatol 2007;19:195–203.

46. Evrard S, Le Moine O, Lazaraki G, et al. Self-expanding plastic stents for benign esophageal lesions. Gastrointest Endosc 2004;60:894–900.

47. Ott C, Ratiu N, Endlicher E, et al. Self-expanding Polyflex plastic stents in esoph-ageal disease: various indications, complications, and outcomes. Surg Endosc 2007;21:889–96.

48. Verschuur EM, Homs MY, Steyerberg EW, et al. A new esophageal stent design (Niti-S stent) for the prevention of migration: a prospective study in 42 patients. Gastrointest Endosc 2006;63:134–40.

49. Verschuur EM, Repici A, Kuipers EJ, et al. New design esophageal stents for the palliation of dysphagia from esophageal or gastric cardia cancer: a randomized trial. Am J Gastroenterol 2008;103:304–12.

50. Bethge N, Sommer A, Vakil N. Treatment of esophageal fistulas with a new polyurethane-covered, self-expanding mesh stent: a prospective study. Am J Gastroenterol 1995;90:2143–6.

51. Do YS, Song HY, Lee BH, et al. Esophagorespiratory fistula associated with esophageal cancer: treatment with a Gianturco stent tube. Radiology 1993;187:673–7.

52. Carazzone A, Bonavina L, Segalin A, et al. Endoscopic palliation of oesophageal cancer: results of a prospective comparison of Nd:YAG laser and ethanol injection. Eur J Surg 1999;165:351–6.

53. Carter R, Smith JS, Anderson JR. Palliation of malignant dysphagia using the Nd:YAG laser. World J Surg 1993;17:608–13 [discussion: 14].

54. Litle VR, Luketich JD, Christie NA, et al. Photodynamic therapy as palliation for esophageal cancer: experience in 215 patients. Ann Thorac Surg 2003;76:1687–92 [discussion: 92–3].

55. Lightdale CJ, Heier SK, Marcon NE, et al. Photodynamic therapy with porfimer sodium versus thermal ablation therapy with Nd:YAG laser for palliation of esophageal cancer: a multicenter randomized trial. Gastrointest Endosc 1995;42:507–12.

56. Heier SK, Rothman KA, Heier LM, et al. Photodynamic therapy for obstructing esophageal cancer: light dosimetry and randomized comparison with Nd:YAG laser therapy. Gastroenterology 1995;109:63–72.

57. Sur RK, Donde B, Levin VC, et al. Fractionated high dose rate intraluminal brachytherapy in palliation of advanced esophageal cancer. Int J Radiat Oncol Biol Phys 1998;40:447–53.

58. Sur RK, Levin CV, Donde B, et al. Prospective randomized trial of HDR brachytherapy as a sole modality in palliation of advanced esophageal carcinoma–an International Atomic Energy Agency study. Int J Radiat Oncol Biol Phys 2002;53:127–33.

59. Brewster AE, Davidson SE, Makin WP, et al. Intraluminal brachytherapy using the high dose rate microSelectron in the palliation of carcinoma of the oesophagus. Clin Oncol (R Coll Radiol) 1995;7:102–5.

60. Homs MY, Eijkenboom WM, Coen VL, et al. High dose rate brachytherapy for the palliation of malignant dysphagia. Radiother Oncol 2003;66:327–32.

61. Siersema PD. Treatment options for esophageal strictures. Nat Clin Pract Gastroenterol Hepatol 2008;5:142–52.

62. Homs MY, Steyerberg EW, Eijkenboom WM, et al. Single-dose brachytherapy versus metal stent placement for the palliation of dysphagia from oesophageal cancer: multicentre randomised trial. Lancet 2004;364:1497–504.

63. Sander R, Hagenmueller F, Sander C, et al. Laser versus laser plus afterloading with iridium-192 in the palliative treatment of malignant stenosis of the esophagus: a prospective, randomized, and controlled study. Gastrointest Endosc 1991;37:433–40.

64. Brooks JA, Kesler KA, Johnson CS, et al. Prospective analysis of quality of life after surgical resection for esophageal cancer: preliminary results. J Surg Oncol 2002;81:185–94.

Index

Note: Page numbers of article titles are in **boldface** type.

A

Abdominal obesity, *versus* overall obesity, as risk factor for Barrett's esophagus and cancer, 437–443
Acid exposure, gastroesophageal reflux disease and, role in development of Barrett's esophagus, 396–401
    chronic inflammation, 399–400
    duodenal contents, 399
    epithelial defense mechanisms, 399
    immune factors, 400–401
Acid suppression, for Barrett's esophagus, prevention of cancer by, 503–504
    risk factor for esophageal cancer, 476
Adenocarcinoma, esophageal, early-stage, effective treatment of, 429
    low risk of, with nondysplastic Barrett's esophagus, 426
    medical therapy of Barrett's esophagus in prevention of, **503–508**
    neoadjuvant therapy for, **533–546**
        adjuvant therapy, 533
        chemotherapy, 531–533
        combined chemoradiotherapy, 533–535
            definitive, without surgery, 539
            newer regimens of, 538–539
            phase III trials of, 535–538
        positron emission tomography directed therapy, 539–540
        radiation therapy, 533
    risk factors for development of, **469–485**
        acid suppression, 476
        age, 472
        alcohol consumption, 474
        antireflux surgery, 476
        Barrett's esophagus, 467–471, 521–522
            biomarkers, 470–471
            dysplasia, 469–470
            segment length, 468–469
        diet, 475
        drugs that relax lower esophageal sphincter, 476
        family history, 472–473
        gender, 472
        Helicobacter pylori, 474
        NSAIDs and aspirin, 475
        obesity, 440–441, 473–474
        race, 472
        reflux symptoms and esophagitis, 471–472
        smoking, 474

Surg Oncol Clin N Am 18 (2009) 561–571
doi:10.1016/S1055-3207(09)00050-7
1055-3207/09/$ – see front matter © 2009 Elsevier Inc. All rights reserved.

surgonc.theclinics.com

Moving?

Make sure your subscription moves with you!

To notify us of your new address, find your **Clinics Account Number** (located on your mailing label above your name), and contact customer service at:

E-mail: elspcs@elsevier.com

800-654-2452 (subscribers in the U.S. & Canada)
314-453-7041 (subscribers outside of the U.S. & Canada)

Fax number: 314-523-5170

Elsevier Periodicals Customer Service
11830 Westline Industrial Drive
St. Louis, MO 63146

*To ensure uninterrupted delivery of your subscription, please notify us at least 4 weeks in advance of move.